A HISTORY OF ORTHOPEDICS

By
Justin Howland, M.D.

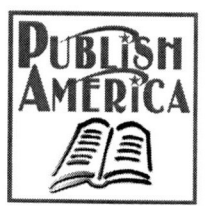

PublishAmerica
Baltimore

© 2011 by Justin Howland, M.D.
All rights reserved. No part of this book may be reproduced, stored in a retrieval system or transmitted in any form or by any means without the prior written permission of the publishers, except by a reviewer who may quote brief passages in a review to be printed in a newspaper, magazine or journal.

First printing

PublishAmerica has allowed this work to remain exactly as the author intended, verbatim, without editorial input.

Hardcover 978-1-4626-0277-3
Softcover 978-1-4626-0278-0
PUBLISHED BY PUBLISHAMERICA, LLLP
www.publishamerica.com
Baltimore

Printed in the United States of America

The reader is advised that this history is not intended to be comprehensive, but will of necessity omit many orthopedic personages who have done much to forward the development of orthopedic surgery as it exists today. For a more complete history please refer to the text of Leonard Peltier, M.D. listed in the bibliography. Much of the material for this book was gathered by the late S. Arthur Frankel, M.D. Discrepancies in dates or deeds found in this essay reflect the great variation which different authors put in the literature.

Thanks go to John Lange, M.D. for his assistance in the preparation of this manuscript.

This book is dedicated to Tracy and Becky.

CHAPTER 1
Ancient Times

Many thousand years before the concept of the specialist in diseases of the bones and joints evolved, men began to use some of the tools, and later the principles, on which the specialty of orthopedic surgery is founded. Written history began about 5000 years ago, but factual recorded knowledge of medicine had its beginning in the Valley of the Nile prior to the years 3200 B.C., when the first of the Egyptian dynasties began. The Egyptians had perfected the science of embalming, and as early as 2700 B.C., functional splints were found on the bodies of cadavers. For almost the next 2000 years, medicine remained more pervaded by mysticism and superstition than it was distinguished by any real effort of scientific investigation.

The beginning of scientific medicine came with the Greeks, with the great Alexandrian anatomists of the third century B.C., and the physicians of the day who recorded all factual medical knowledge of their time in a monumental series of texts known as the Corpus Hippocraticum. Hippocrates was the first to separate the practice of medicine from the traditions of superstition, religion, and magic, and to base it on a careful study of nature. Although he actually wrote a small portion of the seventy-odd books ascribed to him, the Corpus stood for 500 years as the basis for all medical knowledge. Two of these books were on "The Articulations" and "On Fractures", neither of which was written by Hippocrates. The surgeons at the time were well aware of such things as contractures, atrophy of disuse and decubitus ulcers. There was nothing laudable about pus, and they made every effort to maintain cleanliness, did dressing changes frequently and advocated rest for injured parts. Devices of wood and iron were used for limbs as early as

400 B.C., and they devised a rather crude method for treating recurrent dislocation of the shoulder, not too dissimilar in principle, at least, from some of the repairs attempted today. They attempted to limit external rotation by scarifying the lax part of the capsule. A cautery was introduced through the axilla to effect their "imbrications". Congenital dislocation of the hip was known, but treatment was not manipulative. (This did not come until the 19th Century.) Traction was applied by tying the patient's feet to the ceiling while an attendant hung on them. The Scamnum Hippocrates was a machine for increasing the traction, and was essentially a windlass which could exert tremendous pull on the affected part.

As Christianity appeared, and the influence of Greece declined, it was Rome which became the leader in the field of medical progress. Under the Pharaohs of Egypt, the deformed and crippled were destroyed whenever possible. Humanitarianism was introduced by Hippocrates and reached its zenith in the person of Christ. It was not until hundreds of years later, however, that society became aware of its responsibilities to the physically handicapped and provided material help for them. Of the many Romans such as Antyllas (A.D. 200), who advocated tenotomy for contractures, and Aurelianus (A.D. 400), who used passive movement and splints for paralysis, Galen (A.D. 131-201) was the man whose influence and teachings outstripped all others. In spite of the fact that many of his concepts were erroneous and perpetuated for around 600 years by the tremendous stature that the man had, he was a brilliant man who made some real contributions to medicine. While many of his colleagues were talking in terms of "animal humours, vital principles, and life spirit", Galen wrote of the neuromuscular control of voluntary musculature and the independent contractility thereof. He believed the brain to be the central regulating force for the neuromuscular system and while he was distinguishing venous from arterial blood, others of his time still believed they carried "animal humours". He was the first to use the terms "kyphosis, lordosis, and scoliosis". Galen believed in the teachings of Hippocrates, both practicing them and expanding them.

CHAPTER 2
Greco-Roman Times

It was Greco-Roman medicine, essentially unchanged from the time of Galen and Hippocrates, that dominated the civilized world until the Great Awakening which occurred in the 12th century. This foretold the end of medieval times and the beginning of the renaissance in the 13th century. With the decline of Rome, which began in the third century A.D., the Arabians rapidly became a highly developed people, but Mohammed and the Koran forbade dissection and the killing of animals, so little was done to change what had already existed for years as far as medical progress was concerned. Civilized people still looked upon the cripple as something to be abhorred. In Europe the dwarf was so popular as a court jested that parents deliberately maimed their young for the prices they might bring at court.

In spite of the fact that Greco-Roman medicine was still in vogue, its essence had been diluted and altered by the many men who had followed the "Hippocratic method" using their own concept of what it precisely entailed. A good philosophical summary of the Corpus was set forth by Paul of Aegina (A.D. 625-690), and it helped to perpetuate the medicine of Hippocrates and Galen. The Hippocratic method was tried, but if it failed, the art of the times such as "suitable applications of olive oil, pigeon dung, snake oil and other essences" were used. Such was the rather stagnant state of medicine until the 12th century when the great universities of Europe were being founded.

CHAPTER 3
From the 12th to the 17th century

King Roger of Sicily in 1140 was the first to require certification for the practice of medicine. In 1110 the University of Paris was founded, followed by Bologna in 1113, Oxford in 1167, Montpellier in 1181, Padua in 1222 and Naples in 1224. At the medical center in Salerno, which was the first European center of medical learning, great stress was placed on the study of anatomy. At Bologna the study of anatomy was further advanced, especially after the year 1240 when the Emperor Frederick II permitted and compelled dissection in the Italian medical schools. Also at Bologna much was done to rid the world of thousands of years of accumulated debris in terms of bulky, cumbersome splints and braces, replacing them with simpler, lighter devices. Their work culminated with Paré, in the modern art of brace-making. Guy de Chuliac (1300-1368) was Professor of Surgery at Montpellier, in France, and was the chief representative of medieval surgery. He was a great historian and teacher who devised the traction-suspension method for treatment of femoral fractures.

By the end of the 16th century there were more great names in medicine than I could name in an hour. Some of the more outstanding people and their contribution can be listed later, but first there are several things that began to take place at this time which can best be discussed apart from the influence of any given individual. From the time of Hippocrates orthopedics had been a craft, and its craftmen were manipulators and appliance-fitters. In Homer's time the surgeon was an "iatros"—a remover of arrows. Although his status had somewhat improved in the ensuing years, it was not until the 16th century with the work of John Hunter and Ambrose Paré that anything significant was done to elevate the barber-surgeon to professional status. Another seemingly unrelated event which was to have profound influence on the future of orthopedics was the invention in 1346 of cannon shot, and prior to this in 1331, the use of firearms. These were to produce a host of skeletal injuries and with them the need for men trained in their treatment. Around 1450 movable type printing made available to large numbers of physicians information which had previously been much more restricted in circulation. Many of the old texts and classics of medical literature were printed and spread throughout the civilized world. Society was becoming aware of its responsibilities to its disabled when in 1601 the English Parliament passed its Poor Relief Act—the first specific effort at care for the disabled.

Beginning with Leonardo da Vinci (1452-1519) and ending with Vesalius, the anatomy of the human body became a living, dynamic, functional science. Da Vinci was a master anatomist who had more understanding of musculoskeletal dynamics than anyone who had preceded him. Vesalius (1514-1564) who worked at Padua in Italy, compiled his "De Fabrica Humani Corporis" which was published in 1543, and this showed him to be the greatest anatomist of his time. Ambrose Paré (1510-1590) was the end-product of the renaissance in surgery. He was a man of tremendous political power and prestige. Paré humanized surgery of his day by advocating ligature for amputations to replace the customary hot oil used to obtain hemostasis. He used the tourniquet and ligature for amputation, devised many braces, prostheses, and he dignified the barber-surgeons of France like no other had before him. It was with Paré that modern medicine truly had its beginning.

Although there were many outstanding men working in the field of medicine between 1590 and 1728 when John

Hunter was born, it was Hunter who was next to exert a truly profound influence on the medical thinking of his time and of subsequent times. As a young man John was sent to Glasgow to study cabinet-making, but persuaded his brother, William, to accept him as an assistant in anatomy. Although William was a brilliant man, and published a good treatise on the nutrition of articular cartilage, his image is pale in comparison to that left by his younger brother. More will be written about John Hunter in a moment, but between the death of Paré and the birth of Hunter much had been accomplished, and at least something need be said about it.

William Harvey (1578-1657), a man who obtained his doctorate in medicine both at Padua and later at Cambridge, published his "de motu cordis et sanguinis" in 1628, shattering Galenic concepts of the circulation for all time. Had Anton van Leeuwenhoek (1632-1723) been born 50 years earlier, Harvey might have answered his final question—that of how the arterial circulation got back into the veins. Without the microscope he could not see the capillaries, as did Marcello Malphigi (1628-1694) in 1660. Giovanni Borelli (1608-1697) was an Italian physicist and astronomer who is said to be the founder of modern kinetics. His iatrophysical school explained bodily motion in terms of physics, rather than chemistry. He gave his views in "De Motu Animalium". Tenotomy, advocated as early as 200 A.D., was done for the first time in 1685 by Isacius Minius on a child with wry neck. Clopton Havers, from 1689-1601, gave a series of lectures to the Royal Society. These were later published as the "Osteologia Nova", in which was contained the first adequate description of the histologic appearance of bones and joints.

CHAPTER 4
The 18th Century

Orthopedically speaking, there were two outstanding events which took place in the 18th century. Nicholas Andry in 1741 published his "Orthopedia" and in so doing, coined the term. He was the professor of medicine at the University of Paris and wrote extensively on curvature of the spine. Jean-Andre Venel, a Geneva physician, in 1790 established a hospital for skeletal deformities at Orbe, Switzerland. It was essentially a non-surgical hospital devoted to the care of deformed children, but it was, nevertheless, a true orthopedic hospital with treatment of skeletal deformity as its primary concern. It was also about this time that a controversy began which was to last for around a century.

Albrecht von Haller, an 18th century physiologist, studied the formation of bone and came up with the theory that the arteries of bone were the source of all osteogenesis. Henri Louis Duhamel reported that it was only the cambium layer of the periosteum which produced bone. The argument raged back and forth until it was known internationally. It was ended by John Goodsir (1814-1876) of Edinburgh when he demonstrated that osteoid was formed by cells, called osteoblasts. In Italy Galvanni and Volta were experimenting with electrophysiology. Peter Camper (1722-1790) wrote a very lucid book on the anatomy and dynamic physiology of the foot from which most subsequent studies originated. This was also the day of Percival Pott (1714-1788). In 1768 Pott published his essay on fractures and dislocations. Although spinal tuberculosis carries his name in the form of Pott's Disease to this day, he described only the deformity and the sequelae, not its pathogenesis or even its tuberculous nature. Of all the men in the 18th century who advanced the cause of the surgeon, none did more than John Hunter (1728-1793).

Hunter was a productive man who thought deeply about the things he said, wrote prodigiously on diseases of bones and joints, pseudarthosis, mechanism of repair of fractures, inflammation, tendon repair and the dynamic nature of bone. He based all of his teachings on the principle that "the only rational means of treatment are those which are based on the natural recuperative power of the body". He placed a great deal of emphasis on the host's reaction to disease. Particularly because of his ability and partially because of his power to influence those about him, Hunter became a powerful figure in medicine in the latter half of the 18th century. According to Bick, it was with him that the modern period in orthopedics began.

CHAPTER 5
The 19th Century—Orthopedics in England

With the coming of the 19th century the names of the people active in orthopedic endeavors numbers in the hundreds. In an effort to keep within the scope of this book I have had to do two things. Firstly, I have had to limit my discussion almost exclusively to those men who changed the direction and purpose of orthopedics, rather than add technical improvements. Secondly, I have left the discussion of orthopedics in America as a separate topic, to be discussed individually and not concurrent with the inquiry into things as they were taking place on the continent.

At the beginning of the 19th century, the treatment of fractures was just about what it had been for over 200 years. It was Hugh Owen Thomas (1843-1891) who changed the whole concept of orthopedics, both technically and socially. Thomas himself, however, didn't live to see this. Perhaps the best characterization of the man was written by McMurray of Liverpool: "Thomas wrote with difficulty, printed his own books, which were not for sale, and quarreled with his contemporaries and readers on almost every page". He wrote in the narrative, paid no heed whatsoever to statistics and found fault with virtually everyone. Thomas may never have bothered to publish anything at all if Rushton Parker, who was associated with him, hadn't persuaded him to do so.

Thomas' father, and his father before him, had been bonesetters in Liverpool. Hugh Owen Thomas learned what he could from his father, but then went to Edinburgh to become certified in medicine. (In 1858 professional status was conferred upon physicians.) Early in his career he fully grasped the teaching of an earlier English surgeon, John Hilton, that rest, properly used, was a curative. He spent his whole active life at 11 Nelson Street, where he had his office and a complete brace shop. Aside from being a master at the construction and fitting of various appliances, he felt that he alone really understood how to use them. He had a real flair for showmanship, as evidenced by his two-horse rig with scarlet body and bright red wheels. He was never without a cap, coat, gloves, and cigarette. He was so possessive about his methods that he built into some of his devices a fastener which he would seal with wax, then stamp with his signet ring to insure no tampering would be done in his absence. Most of what he earned, he gave away, but he insisted on being paid because "human nature values what it pays for". His passion for work and craftsmanship was intense—he would breakfast at 7:30, see patients until noon, then do 26 operations between lunch and 9:00 o'clock. In his Sunday free clinic he would see about 7000 patients each year. He spoke in terms of "soundness and unsoundness" of limbs and joints. An "unsound" limb or joint was one which was acutely inflamed or in which an active process of disease was taking place. His treatment depended on what disease he was treating and on what stage of its natural history it was in. His principle of "rest, enforced, uninterrupted and prolonged" he applied skillfully, according to what would best suit his patient at the time, and his objectives were long term, rather than simple alleviation of pain. In the true sense of the word, Thomas was a scientist and based his beliefs on what was observable, reproducible and predictable according to the traditional scientific method of hypothesis founded on observation. He was adamant, albeit argumentative, in the assertion of his principles and a master craftsman when it came to applying them. Thomas never set in print precisely what he meant by "rest", but Winnet Orr defined it as he felt Thomas would have. According to Orr, "Rest is that state of a diseased or injured part in which there is never enough motion, or irritation of any other kind, to cause pain, muscle spasm, interference with nerve supply or circulation, or disturbance of the function, local or general, involved in healing and repair". Although Thomas had not the personality to give to the world directly what he had to offer, this was ably done by Robert Jones in England and John Ridlon in America.

Before writing of Sir Robert Jones, I am going to list important men of that era since it is important to know that they contributed to the development of orthopedics.

Rudolph Virchow (1821—1902)—professor of pathology in the University of Berlin.

Crawford Long (1815—1878)—gave ether anesthetic in 1842.

Louis Pasteur (1827—1895)—professor of chemistry, bacteriology, physics and geology. Produced anthrax, cholera, and rabies vaccines. His germ theory led to pasteurization.

Joseph Lister (1827—1912)—in 1867 he announced his principle of wound antisepsis. His dressings consisted of carbolic acid and shellac spread on calico and painted with gutta-percha dissolved in benzene.

Julius Wolff (1836—1910)—"Every change in the form and the function of a bone, or of its function alone, is followed by certain definite changes in its internal architecture and equally definite secondary alterations in its mathematical laws."

Wilhelm Röntgen (1845—1923)—a German physicist who on 8 November 1895 produced and detected electromagnetic radiation in a wavelength range today known as x-rays. For this he was awarded the Nobel Prize for Physics in 1901.

Robert Koch (1843—1910)—at Hamburg, Germany in 1882 he looked at and realized the nature of the tubercle bacillus. He received the Nobel Prize for Medicine in 1905.

A HISTORY OF ORTHOPEDICS

To return to the narrative, Sir Robert Jones (1857—1933) of Liverpool was important in orthopedics. It was fortunate that a man of his stature should come along at a time when so much had already been established. With the contemporaneous advances in the sciences, anesthesia, aseptic technique and x-rays, the time was ripe for someone to establish orthopedic surgery as a specialty. In Belgium and France general surgeons who devoted themselves to the surgery of the growing period were the orthopedists of the day. The Germans were much more mechanical minded and devoted themselves to treatment of injuries and deformities. They cared little about and did little surgery. It was the special interest general surgeons who were the forerunners of the orthopedic surgeons.

It was Robert Jones' uncle, Hugh Owen Thomas, who introduced him to orthopedic practice. At the age of fifteen Jones was working with and helping his uncle in his clinic on Nelson Street. Before reaching the age of thirty his writings had been translated into French, Spanish, and German. As a young surgeon he volunteered for the position of consulting surgeon to the construction of the Manchester Ship Canal in Great Britain. While serving in this capacity he established he first fracture service to care for the injuries incurred on the job. While the irascibility of Thomas made it very difficult for his colleagues to accept his principles, the enormous personal charm and appeal of Jones allowed him to popularize Thomas' concepts as his uncle never could have had he lived a hundred years longer than he did. He was among the first in Britain to utilize the newly discovered x-ray. When World War I began, it gave great impetus to the knowledge of fractures and skeletal injuries. It was Jones who was instrumental in the organization and establishment of the military orthopedic hospitals. He so popularized the subject of orthopedics that following the war, many young men were attracted to the field.

An interesting and famous relationship grew up between Jones and a woman from Shropshire whose name was Agnes Hunt. Agnes was one of 10 children of a Victorian eccentric. From childhood she had crippling joint disease of her hip, probably of a tuberculous nature. This didn't prevent her from training as a nurse, however, and she went on to become the founder of orthopedic nursing in England. That she inherited some of the eccentricity of her mother was apparent in that she owned a horse called "Bacillus" and a dog named "Germ". She and her mother moved into an ancient home in Baschurch, England, and began taking in and caring for crippled children in about the year 1900. She would periodically take her brood to Robert Jones' free clinic for care. On one occasion she saw him herself because of her hip problem. Eventually, she asked him if he wouldn't be the visiting consultant in surgery at her hospital. Apparently the absurdity of the situation struck Jones' fancy, for he promptly accepted. Shortly thereafter, under candlelight in the living room, he did his first operation. Although the beginnings may have been humble and crude, the hospital grew to over 300 beds, was used as a center for military surgery during the war, and then moved to Oswestry in 1921 to become the Robert Jones-Agnes Hunt Orthopedic Hospital. The rather peculiar alliance between these two, who had in common a profound feeling for the need of England's crippled children, became a powerful one. Through their efforts the public also became aware of this need. Legislation followed, charitable groups sprang up, hospitals and clinics were built, and the people of England recognized and accepted their responsibility.

To discuss Jones' contributions as a surgeon would be interesting, but it was his position as a champion of orthopedic surgery as a specialty which was most outstanding. He brought compassion, dignity, and humility into the field as no one before or after him has done. The warmth and affection which people had for him is truly inspiring. On his 70th birthday a "Birthday Volume" of orthopedics was published, containing original articles by the outstanding orthopedists of the day. In it Lord Moynihan wrote, "The story of the triumph of Robert Jones as prophet, high priest and practitioner of orthopedic surgery makes plain the reason for our deep respect. Our affection for him transcends, if it is possible, our gratitude for his professional worthiness. Few men have ever possessed in so radiant a degree the genius for friendship. No one can be long in his company, no one can work with him or play with him, without realizing the sweet simplicity of his character, and the greatness of his heart. He speaks ill of no man. He seeks and finds good in all things and in all men. He sets an ideal and a standard of action in friendship which all strive to reach when with him". When he died in 1933, he was mourned by thousands.

One of Jones' contemporaries was Arbuthnot Lane (1856—1943). He was a British surgeon who was deeply impressed by the germ theory of sepsis. During the earlier days when general surgeons were treating bones and joints with the same finesse as they did in the peritoneal cavity, the quotation was passed about that "bone is filled not with good red marrow, but with black ingratitude". Lane was a scrupulous advocate, not of antisepsis, but of asepsis. He was well aware of the fact that the powerful concoctions surgeons were dumping into operative wounds were killing about as many cells as they were organisms. His "no touch" technique was as tedious as it was scrupulous, but there was one thing about it which gave it distinction—it worked. He used sterile caps, gowns, and masks for operating room wear. All of his sponges, swabs, and dressings were sterilized. Instruments were boiled, and he discarded his skin knife. Nothing that was to enter the wound was touched by hand, and his instruments had long handles to keep fingers out. Even his drill bits were re-boiled after each drill hole was made. H.A.T. Fairbank, his pupil, followed and taught his technique with fervor. Fairbank was the first orthopedist in charge of a surgical department with no other responsibilities. When E.C. Wallis was promoted from orthopedic surgeon to full surgeon at Charing Cross Hospital in 1906, there were no further vacancies on the general surgical staff. It was thus that Fairbank became a full-time orthopedic surgeon. Fairbank's atlas on "General Affections of the Skeleton" was considered to be one of the best scientific contributions of the century. (Published in 1951)

In 1896 A.H. Tubby published his text on orthopedic surgery. This was a monumental work in which he stressed the fact that orthopedics was "the surgery of the entire locomotor apparatus". The book did a lot to increase British prestige in orthopedics.

CHAPTER 6
Orthopedics on the continent

Another man who did as much to stress the rehabilitative aspect of orthopedics as Jones was Konrad Biesalski (1863—1930) of Germany. Aside from the pioneer work on tendon transfers that he and Leo Mayer of New York did, he established the first rehab center in Europe. As late as 1913 the general surgeons in Germany were still doing almost all of the bone and joint surgery. The orthopedists in teaching centers were given the privilege of doing subcutaneous tenotomies, though. Because of this practice Biesalski had established a large crippled children's hospital in Berlin. After World War I his hospital was converted into a rehab center, and was established prior to Robert Jones' center at Shepherd's Bush.

Adolph Lorenz (1854—1946), famous for introducing the bifurcation osteotomy, had such an enormous clinic in Vienna that he and his associates had to find shortcuts to handle the patient load. One such example that Leo Mayer described was as follows: In the treatment of tuberculosis of the hip, three visits were required. On the first the patient was placed in a single hip spica cast. He was told to return in one year with the expectation that his flexion-adduction contracture would have become solidly ankylosed. On the second visit, a subcutaneous osteotomy was done, a second hip spica was applied, and the next appointment given for 6 months. When this amount of time had elapsed, and the osteotomy was solid, the cast was removed, and the patient was discharged.

In 1928 Axhausen, the German pathologist, published his epic monograph on the pathologic anatomy of free bone transplants. He gave the name "schleichender Ersatz" to something no one before him had ever described—the replacement of dead graft bone by living, newly formed bone. It was Phemister's translation by which the term became known in this country—creeping substitution.

There was an old Olivetan monastery on a hill near the outskirts of Bologna, Italy. Francesco Rizzoli, one time professor of surgery at the University of Bologna, bought the monastery in 1880 and left his entire fortune as an endowment to the orthopedic hospital which he created there. The Rizzoli Institute thus founded became a favored destination for orthopedic surgeons from all over the world. By 1920 Vittoria Putti (1880—1920), the third director of the institute, was doing arthroplasties, femoral lengthening, bone grafts, kineplastic operations (functional modeling of amputated stumps) and many other surgical procedures. But the thing for which he was most famous was his work on congenital dislocation of the hip. At that time in northern Italy more children were being born with CDH than anywhere else in the world. Putti studied them clinically, anatomically and pathologically. His publications on the subject are classics, but his greatest contribution was that of preventive orthopedics. He decided that a lot of trouble could be averted if infants were diapered in extension, and suggested that each of them be x-rayed. He was one of the most outstanding early 20th century orthopedists, and it is likely that his work on CDH will be the source of enduring fame.

Other famous continental orthopedists include Stromeyer, Little, Paget, Lexer, Macewen, Brodie, Ollier, Syme and others who contribute significantly to surgical progress in the late 19th and early 20th centuries. In Europe the story of the emancipation of the orthopedic surgeon had come a long way by the beginning of the 20th century. The arrow pullers, bonesetters and barber-surgeons had ceased to exist, and many men skilled in the practice of bone and joint surgery were expanding the scope and direction of our knowledge almost daily. The image of the orthopedist as a surgeon, rather than a manipulator or bracer was becoming established. The evolution of European orthopedics had a strong influence on the direction of American orthopedics.

CHAPTER 7
Orthopedics in North America—the 18th century

In 1607, the year of Jamestown's establishment, modern medicine had barely gotten started on the continent with the work of Paré and Vesalius. This was 134 years before the name Orthopedics, let alone the practice thereof, was to be conceived. So as far as the development of the specialty was concerned, we were not far behind. With the establishment of Harvard in 1636 and Yale in 1701, North America had its first two centers of higher education, but it wasn't until 1765 that the first medical school in Philadelphia began. Prior to this and for some time thereafter, the common law of the land was that anyone who felt so qualified could legally practice medicine. There was liability for any damage one might do, but consent for treatment was the only license required. As was the custom in Europe, those few who did make an attempt at formal training did so by the apprentice method. This consisted of a period of about 7 years during which time one faithfully attended the man who was the master. Since there was grave doubt about the qualification of these masters, it is easy to understand why the early colonists turned to their public officials and the ministry for medical aid. Quacks and charlatans abounded, and of the 3500 practitioners of medicine in the country 155 years after the Plymouth landing, only 400 had their degree in medicine. The only decent education in medicine was derived from men who had gone to Europe for their training, then returned to America to act as private tutors, usually in anatomy. The first effort at curtailing "do-it-yourself medicine" came in 1760, when the state of New York passed a law requiring a license to practice. Shortly thereafter, state medical societies began to form and took over the job of licensure. When John Morgan (1735—1789), who had trained in Edinburgh, came home in 1765, he was granted the position of Professor of the Theory and Practice of Physick at the College of Philadelphia. William Shippen became the Professor of Anatomy and Surgery, and the first medical school in the country had its rather humble beginnings. It graduated the first class on June 2, 1768—ten students were given their M.B. (This followed the English custom of first granting a bachelor's degree, then allowing the candidates to attain their doctorate in two to three years on the basis of a thesis which they had to publically give and defend.) The second school was established in New York in 1767 at Kings College (later to become Columbia), and the third followed at Harvard in 1782. Dartmouth medical school opened its doors in 1798, and the several hundred foreign-trained American doctors in the country prior to 1800 were about to be joined by many American-trained colleagues.

CHAPTER 8
19TH Century—Philadelphia

American Medicine was getting on its feet during the time when orthopedics was going through its period of tenotomy and subcutaneous surgery. (1780—1880) It was the belief of the times that air was the cause of suppuration, and the subcutaneous operation was designed to allow as little of the ambient air as possible into the wound. Whether or not the orthopedist should do any surgery, however, was a matter of far greater interest to the men who were establishing the specialty. The term "orthopedic surgery" first appeared in print in a book by Valentine Mott in 1841. As was generally the case in those days, Mott was a general surgeon (most famous for his vascular surgery), but he did a certain amount of orthopedic surgery as well. However, among the men who considered themselves orthopedists, the course the specialty was to take was not at all clear. In Philadelphia the influence of John Hunter was widely transmitted to America in the person of Phillip Syng Physick (1768—1837). The University of Pennsylvania was established by Benjamin Franklin in 1740. Physick graduated from this university, and in 1789 went to London to become house surgeon to John Hunter at St. George's hospital. He took his M.D. from Edinburgh at age 24, and despite Hunter's efforts to induce him to remain in Europe, he returned to Philadelphia and went on to become its first professor of surgery in 1805. Hunter's principle of rest in fractures and joint disease was apparent in Physick's teaching. It was the former's "principle of stimulation" that led Physick to pass a seton through an ununited humeral shaft fracture and obtain union in five months. After he gave up the chair of surgery for that of anatomy in 1816, he experimented with animal tissues as a suture material. He became the first man in America to use absorbable suture, made of horsehide, deerskin and parchment. One of Physick's pupils, Dr. Rhea Barton (1794—1871) was said to have done the first intertrochanteric osteotomy in the country. The patient was a sailor with a 90° flexion contracture of the hip. According to Barton, "the operation was done in seven minutes and not one blood vessel had to be secured". Barton felt the operation was a success, in spite of the fact that the man ended up with no motion in his hip—an unhappy circumstance that, as Barton put it, was due to "habits of intemperance,…this, with all its train of evils, abuse of health was, no doubt, the cause of the change which afterwards took place in the artificial joint."

CHAPTER 9
19TH Century—New York

Among the men who were admittedly general surgeons, doing general (including orthopedic) surgery, there were no problems as to the nature of their practice. Their right to surgery of all kinds had not yet been threatened, nor would it be until the end of the 19th century. Those who considered themselves orthopedists, however, had much with which to concern themselves. When William Detmold (1808—1899) came from Hanover to New York in 1837 to become surgeon to Bellevue Hospital in 1841, he brought with him the approved orthopedic methods of Germany, and his teacher, Louis Stromeyer. He was most famous for his evacuation of a brain abscess in 1850, but he did introduce tenotomy to the United States. Another of Stromeyer's pupils, Louis Bauer (1814—1898), came to Brooklyn in 1852 and began lecturing on orthopedic surgery at the Medical and Surgical Institution of Brooklyn. That wasn't all he did, though. While in Europe he had become convinced of the efficacy and good sense of H.O. Thomas' ideas, and because of this he kept up a running commentary of criticism of the "big four" in New York orthopedics—C. F. Taylor, H. G. Davis, L. A. Sayre and James Knight. (Of Bauer, Thomas was quoted as saying, "In my early life I was in my practice a close imitator and ardent admirer of my friend, Dr. Louis Bauer, the best exponent of American orthopedics").

James Knight (1810—1877) was a dogmatic, stubborn, conservative whose initial claim to fame was a truss which he designed for "broken bellies". In order to keep from being bothered by his critics, in 1879 he established the Hospital for Ruptured and Crippled, which he ran with an iron fist for 14 years. He practiced "surgico-mechanics", devised a back brace and wrote a book, *Orthopaedia*. In his hospital he practiced "enforced hygiene, regular and nutritious dietary", and applied bracing and bandaging to deformities, varicose veins, piles, procedentia uteri and ectopia vesicae. He would not, however, have anything to do with Davis' elastic traction.

Henry G. Davis (1807—1896) was the leading proponent of what he named "elastic traction", which was commonly thought of abroad as the "American" method of treating hip disease. Davis also devised a brace which he felt was so good that he had it patented. The basic principle around which he based all of his treatment was motion without friction. That he was not a surgeon was evident when he published his book in 1867. It contained Hippocrates' quotation: "as a mode of cure it requires neither cutting, nor burning nor any other complex means".

C. Fayette Taylor (1827—1899) was still another of the early New York "orthopedists". He was essentially a physical therapist who had had only one year medical training prior to 1858 when he constructed his "spinal assistant" for supporting tuberculous spines. In 1866 he founded the New York Orthopedic Dispensary, in which he was complete master of his own treatment.

The most commanding figure of the four was Louis A. Sayre (1820—1903). According to Keith he was the forerunner of the modern school of orthopedic surgery. He was one of the founders of Bellevue Hospital Medical College, and it was at this institution that he became the first Professor of Orthopedic Surgery in the country in 1861. Sayre was a man, as were many of his contemporaries, whose enthusiasm was unhampered by exact knowledge. He always insisted he was first of all a general surgeon and for years refused to join the American Orthopedic Association, and never became president, a position held by his son, Reginald, in 1904. As a young trainee, he had opened a cold abscess in a knee against the advice of his superior. He was told, "You damned blockhead, you've killed the man". But the man didn't die, and Sayre "never believed anything that any of them told me after that". He read little, knew nothing about other people's failures, and went blithely along doing well at things he wasn't supposed to be able to do. When younger, he had crossed the continent in a stagecoach, breaking his leg along the way. He directed the driver and did the reduction, using flour paste, strips of cloth and some old copies of the New York Tribune for immobilization. According to Sayre, this was the first good use to which the paper had ever been put. His story of his stay in Salt Lake City is rather amusing. He said that when he got there Brigham Young ordered Hiram Smith to have a vision foretelling of a great surgeon's coming among the Mormon host. In a personal communication he later wrote, "Heber Kimber, one of the leading elders, had eleven squint-eyed children, all of whom I operated, and there were club feet, and wrynecks, and diseases of all sorts, kinds and descriptions, so that I enjoyed my stay very much".

In spite of the obvious fact that these early pioneers of orthopedics had their fair share of human frailties, it is well to consider their deeds in light of the times. According to Holmes, "the atmosphere was vocal with the flippant loquacity of half-knowledge", and indeed it was. Each man was his own authority and medicine lacked the sophistication that it was later to attain. Knight was considered behind the times because he used no elastic extension. Davis felt that all his discoveries had been stolen from him—a little touch of paranoia which earned him the criticism of his contemporaries when he patented his brace. Sayre was called an arrogant and mendacious exploiter of adventurous treatment by the others. Yet in spite of their fighting and almost complete lack of the soundness of judgment of men like Thomas and Hunter, these early men did a lot for the specialty. For one thing, they gave it publicity. Their authoritarianism in the hospitals which they founded left the way clear for their followers to pursue their art unhampered by restrictions. And since in their vanity they were willing to tackle almost any malady, they were gradually tearing down the restrictions which time had imposed on the specialty.

History names Judson, Shaffer, Gibney, and Phelps as the successors to the four pioneers. They lived and worked right in the middle of the "strap and buckle" period and because of this they had a lot to do with the direction orthopedics was to take. Prior to the time that a group of men who considered themselves orthopedists emerged, orthopedic diseases were treated by general surgeons and as such had no question as to whether or not surgery should be a part of their art. Among the early orthopedists, though, the battle over surgery was long and heated, with the establishment of the orthopedist as a surgeon requiring the entire 19th century to transpire. Not the least vocal among the men letting their views be heard was Newton W. Shaffer (1846—1928).

Shaffer trained with Knight at the Hospital for Ruptured and Crippled (later renamed Hospital for Special Surgery), then went to the New York Orthopedic Dispensary where he replaced Taylor as chief. Here he remained for 21 years until he resigned after a fight with the Board of Trustees, going then to Haverstraw where he founded the New York State Reconstruction Hospital. As a propagandist, Shaffer took second place to no one, but he believed orthopedics should be a non-operative specialty and was perhaps the last influential member of the old school who tried to preserve strap-and-bucklism. He was one of the original organizers of the American Orthopedic Association in 1887 and made every effort to lead orthopedists away from operative work because "to mingle surgery and mechanics is to endanger both". Shaffer was an influential man, but he made few friends, and not the least among his enemies was Hugh Owen Thomas.

John Ridlon (1852—1936) had earlier gone to Liverpool to visit Thomas. On his arrival he was quoted as saying, "Mr. Thomas, I am Dr. Ridlon from New York. I have come to Liverpool to find out if your results in the treatment of joint disease are as good as you say they are in your book. I want to know whether I am a fool, or you are a liar". On his return to New York, Ridlon became Shaffer"s assistant (1881) at St. Lukes where the latter had been attending surgeon since 1872. Ridlon had become convinced that Thomas' principles and understanding of disease were greatly superior to anything he had yet seen, so in 1888 when Shaffer became consulting surgeon, and Ridlon took his old job as attending surgeon to St. Lukes, he began using some of Thomas' methods and splints. This was the beginning of a long and heated verbal battle between Ridlon, Shaffer, Thomas, and the Board of Managers of St. Luke's Hospital. Thomas wrote his "Argument with the Censor at St. Luke's hospital, New York" which was actually an indictment of most of the prominent U. S. orthopedists of the day. Thomas was intimately familiar with everything his opponents had said, written or done, and had picked up a lot of inside information from his long talks with Ridlon. As a result, he picked the Americans to pieces, finding every error they made, every failure to give proper credit and every contradiction of previous statements printed. The Medical Board of the hospital actually sided with Ridlon in response to Shaffer's attack, but Shaffer brought his influence to bear on the Board of Managers, and one year after his appointment, Ridlon resigned and was quietly replaced by T. H. Myers. Shaffer won the battle, but lost the war, however. His opposition to Ridlon brought out a lot of the latent disfavor of his contemporaries and culminated in his replacement by one of the prominent and progressive surgeons of the day, Russell Hibbs (1869—1932).

The battle between the strap-and-buckle men and the surgeons continued. Virgil P. Gibney (1847—1927), the acting president of the American Orthopedic Association at its first meeting, had trained with Sayre at Bellevue, then gone on to spend 13 years with Knight at Ruptured and Crippled. When Gibney published his book, "Diseases of the Hip", advocating treatment not in agreement with Knight, his resignation was immediately forthcoming. When Knight died in 1877, Gibney came back as chief. Although Gibney was not much of a surgeon himself, he foresaw the direction of things to come, saying that "the orthopedic surgeon should first be a well-trained surgeon, and then know how to use braces, traction and plaster of paris". Under his direction, the organization and function of Knight's hospital was completely changed to be more in accord with the more progressive orthopedists of the day.

Of the influential men of the time, none had more authority and prestige than John Ridlon (1852—1936). After Shaffer effected his departure from St. Lukes, he tried several places to establish himself, and eventually ended up in Chicago. From there he went on to become a politically powerful leader in the affairs of the American Orthopedic Association as well as in orthopedic education and practice in general throughout the country. He became so wrapped up in the function of the AOA that he was opposed to the formation of the Academy later on. During his life he remained a disciple of Thomas and did a great deal to spread his thoughts and principles throughout the country. He apparently had more in common with Thomas than medical philosophy because he criticized freely what he didn't like, and like Thomas, earned the resentment of many of his colleagues. But Ridlon was generous with himself as well as his ideas and taught many young men in this country what orthopedics was about.

CHAPTER 10
New England

New York was not the only place in this country where the practice of orthopedics was taking form. The first orthopedic hospital in the country was opened in Boston in 1837 by John Ball Brown. After J. B. Brown married the famous John Warren's daughter, their son, Buckminster Brown became the first orthopedic specialist in the city. He took charge of the orthopedic ward at Samaritan Hospital in 1861, the first of its kind in New England. John Warren had done the first shoulder disarticulation in America as early as 1781. Robert Lovett (1859—1924) was an outstanding orthopedic pathologist who became Professor of Orthopedic Surgery at Harvard.

The state of Connecticut was one of the first in which orthopedic surgery was recognized and developed. Surprisingly, one of the reasons this was so was the presence and prominence of a famous family of bonesetters—the Sweets. In England the Holton brothers and John Atkinson were widely known for their treatment of bone and joint injuries. In France the family of Bailleul was known far and wide. Men of science generally looked with distrust at the bonesetters as a group, and in describing their practices Pott said, "They regard bone setting as no matter of science; as a thing which the most ignorant farrier may, with utmost ease, become soon and perfectly master of; nay, that he may receive it from his father and family as a kind of heritage". In the true sense of the word, the New England Sweets were bonesetters, but to a man they were a quiet, unpretentious lot, not interested in exploiting their "secrets" or gaining great wealth. They had the respect of the medical community, and it was their enormous popularity which helped in gaining acceptance for the men who later became trained specialists in the treatment of bone and joint injuries. As a matter of interest, the Sweets did not perish when laws began to restrict the practice of medicine without a license. They rolled with the tide, and many of them went on to get their medical training. John Sweet not only took formal training in medicine, but went on to become a boarded orthopedic surgeon.

CHAPTER 11
The West

Aside from his influence in the AOA, Ridlon was also the unofficial leader of what came to be known as the "Western Bloc" of the AOA. This included men like Moore and Gillette of Minneapolis and St. Paul, Griffeth of Kansas City, Packard of Denver, Sherman of San Francisco, and Steele of St. Louis. Prior to Arthur Steindler, Ridlon was probably the most influential teacher of orthopedics in this country.

In 1848 the war with Mexico was ended by treaty, and New Mexico and California became part of the United States. It was less than forty years after this that Harry Sherman (1854—1921) came to San Francisco to be the first practitioner of orthopedics on the coast. He had trained in New York under Louis Sayre, then went to California in 1885, and became the first to hold the chair of orthopedic surgery at the University of California in 1896. George B. Packard (1852—1928) was another of the early settlers of the west. He had obtained his degree from the University of Vermont in 1874 and associated himself with Gibney and Shaffer in New York before leaving for Colorado because of his health. In 1899 he came to Green Mountain Falls, which he eventually left for a stay in Colorado Springs prior to arriving in Denver. He was the first head of the Department of Orthopedics in what was later to become the University of Colorado School of Medicine. While in Denver he helped with the organization and establishment of the Denver Children's Hospital. James T. Watkins joined Sherman in 1902 and became the chief figure in the organization of the Pacific Coast Orthopedic Association. The first true orthopedic hospital in the west was the Children's Hospital in Seattle, established in 1907. Other early teachers of orthopedics in the west were

R. B. Dillehunt (1866—1953) of Portland who helped in the development of the Shrine Children's Hospitals, and C. F. Eikenbary (1877—1932) of Seattle who was a pupil of Ridlon and Whitman.

CHAPTER 12
Advent of anesthesia and x-rays

By the end of the 19th century many things had happened to shape the future of orthopedics and orthopedists. The development of medicine itself had gone through the age of mysticism and half-knowledge, and a physiologic basis was being established for further progress. The bonesetters had been supplanted because the reason for their existence had ceased to be. Men like Hilton, Hunter and Thomas had established Nature as the prime healer and had clarified the principles whereby men of medicine could best assist her. The field of orthopedics had been broadened from the treatment of deformities in children by a small group of special interest general surgeons to include the treatment of bone and joint injuries and diseases in adults as well. Orthopedists themselves had not completely resolved the problem of surgery versus mechanics, but the trend to include the former was already overwhelmingly apparent. Musculoskeletal disease had come all the way from the machines of Hippocrates, through the hands of the bonesetters, had its time with the subcutaneous tenotomy-osteotomy surgeons, strap-and-buckle mechanics and the era of open operative orthopedics was well on its way before 1900. Of the countless individual events which helped to pave the way, it was the discovery of the cause of sepsis, x-ray and anesthesia which did the most to speed things along.

When the great Scottish surgeon, William Macewen, stood before the International Medical Congress in 1884—a time when the mortality from compound fractures ran as high as 80%—and presented his paper, telling of 1800 osteotomies with no fatalities, and only eight infections, his results staggered the imagination of his audience. He received a standing ovation. When the treatment of open fractures reached what Orr called the "height of absurdity" with the Carrell-Dakin irrigation every two hours, it was orthopedic surgeon, Winnett Orr, who brought reason to bear on the problem by simply debriding his wounds and leaving them alone.

It was Herbert Galloway of Winnipeg who publicly evaluated the Lorenz treatment for congenital dislocation of the hip for what it was: "blind, irrational, and deplorably uncertain in results". While it was true that the advent of anesthesia was the springboard for a host of irrational and needless operations, such has been the case with most great discoveries—the good had to be separated from the bad. Without anesthesia, detailed meticulous surgery had been impossible. Its discovery was of singular importance. The addition of x-ray in the late 1800s altered the whole process of diagnosis and prognosis in regard to orthopedic treatment. The introduction of anesthesia helped considerably.

This was effected on October 16th, 1846 when Henry Bigelow induced T. G. Morton (a dentist) to use ether anesthesia for a general surgical procedure. Thus the end of the 19th century saw the field of orthopedics expanding rapidly. It was to be several more years before Royal Whitman's treatment of femoral neck fractures brought orthopedists solidly into the field of fractures. His success and that of others made it clear that they knew better how to care for fractures than the general surgeons of the day, and it wasn't long before their treatment was a well established part of the orthopedic specialty. By 1900 38 of 67 universities in the country mentioned orthopedics as a field of endeavor apart from general surgery.

Of the 29 papers presented at the first ten years of AOA meetings, 114 dealt with tuberculosis with the majority of the remainder being devoted to club feet, scoliosis, congenital hip disease and rickets. In the treatment of tuberculosis, excision of joints occasionally resulted in fusion, but the concept of arthrodesis had not yet matured. The basis for the modern treatment of TB in part came from the pathology lab of Edward H. Nichols of Harvard. He gave the first scholarly description of the pathology of bone and joint tuberculosis. In 1906 Fred H. Albee, an obscure young surgeon from Maine, successfully arthrodesed a hip for osteoarthritis. In 1909, six years after he had graduated from medical school, he presented his operation before the AOA. From then on Albee, his "glass-stopper" fit and his electric saw, went on to become world famous. By 1916 he had operated and fused over 500 tuberculous spines. His graft surgery branched out to include scoliosis and fractures, and his fame was such that orthopedics in general achieved a little more stature.

CHAPTER 13
The 20th century

In the period after the turn of the century and prior to the onset of World War I, knowledge in the basic sciences proceeded to amass at a gratifying rate. Communities began to develop a sense of responsibility for their cripples, and the concept of rehabilitation was becoming a clear one. The decision to change from "Transactions" to "The American Journal of Orthopedic Surgery" in 1903 was more than just a change in names. The Journal now included contributions from non-members, and abstracts of literature from all over the world were added. The inclusion of adults as orthopedic patients opened the way for addition of new information about a host of problems that didn't usually involve children. There developed an interest in back problems, and Goldthwait and Hibbs were among the earliest to write on the subject. Numerous individuals published papers by the hundreds on an almost equal number of subjects. Codman (who was later to begin the Registry of Bone Sarcomas), in 1906 began writing on the painful shoulder. The first AOA symposium on arthritis was held in 1912. Attempts to mobilize ankylosed joints began with a report in 1906 by William Baer of chromicized pig bladder arthroplasty. The emphasis on clinical orthopedics now shared as equal interest with the experimental, of which Abel Phelps' attempt to graft a dog bone—complete with vascular supply—into a child by strapping the two together was one of the more ostentatious examples. In 1901 Whitman's paper on astragalectomy appeared, followed in 1911 by Hoke's work on the pathology and treatment of severe club feet. In 1916 Mayer's papers on tendon transfer began to appear, with the first of Smith-Peterson's revolutionary articles on the treatment of hip fractures appearing the next year. With the onset of war in Europe in 1914, the practice of orthopedics was about to receive its biggest boost of the century. Aside from the invaluable experiences gained by the hundreds of men who had an opportunity to treat and observe the casualties of war, as E. G. Brackett stated in his 1917 address to the Boston Orthopedic Society, the war "had consolidated the ultimate purpose of orthopedic surgery...restoration of function". Following Galloway's denouncement of the Lorenz method, the concept of gentleness in treating hip disease in children flowered. Shelf procedures by Dickson, Gill, Phemister, Compere, and Ober began to appear in the early 1930s, and gradually the indication for open reduction was becoming the failure of an attempt at closed. It was also the 1930s when disc protrusion began to be recognized as an entity. Bunnell's papers based on work done earlier by Mayer and Biesalski, began to appear in 1918, with the establishment of atraumatic technique as the basis for successful hand surgery. The number of significant contributions of the first half of the 20th century is large, and the list of men working in the field is long, but the important thing is that it was in the first part of this century that orthopedic surgery as a separate specialty became firmly established. During that same time the practitioners of the specialty for the first time ceased to argue about what they were going to do. The only point of contention was what was the best way to perform the operation.

CHAPTER 14
Organizing Orthopedics in the United States

When the American Orthopedic Association was organized in 1887, of the fourteen men present, only ten felt the need of an Orthopedic Society. During the next 25 years more and more felt that some type of organization was necessary, and more groups began to form. Orthopedic societies and associations grew up in every major area of the country, but the next major step came in 1912 when Albert H. Freiberg of Cincinnati organized the Orthopedic Section of the American Medical Association. On October 11, 1931 Willis Campbell of Memphis had an unofficial meeting of a few AOA members in Chicago, to discuss the possibility of the formation of a new society of orthopedists. Since the membership in AOA was initially limited to 100, there were quite a few men who began to think of AOA as a type of private club, and the idea of a more inclusive body began to form. In January 1933 at a meeting of the Clinical Orthopedic Society, the American Academy of Orthopedic Surgeons was formally organized, with E. W. Ryerson as the first president. The Academy has become the preeminent provider of musculoskeletal education to orthopedic surgeons and others in the world. Its continuing medical education (CME) activities include a world-renowned Annual Meeting, multiple CME courses held around the country and at the Orthopedic Learning Center, and various medical and scientific publications and electronic media materials.

It wasn't until after the AOA, AMA Section on Orthopedics and the Academy met in 1934 that the American Board of Orthopedic Surgery, Incorporated was formed and membership in the Academy did not require Board certification until 1937. Prior to that the ABOS provided in the articles of incorporation for the evaluation of hospitals and medical schools that were education young surgeons to become orthopedic surgeons. By 1936 the ABOS published formal requirements for certification which stipulated that a candidate—1) must be a graduate of a medical school approved by the AMA Council of Medical Education and Hospitals. 2) must be of high ethical and professional standing. 3) must be duly authorized to practice medicine in the state or province of his residence. 4) must be a member of the AMA or other society approved by the AMA Council of Medical Education and Hospitals. 5) after 1938 must have three years of concentrated instruction in orthopedic surgery approved and acceptable to the ABOS. and 6) must have two years further experience in the actual practice of orthopedic surgery and also have knowledge of the basic medical sciences related to orthopedic surgery. Thus, the first formal educational standards were established for orthopedic surgery in the United States.

The Audio-Visual program of the Academy was organized in 1939, and in 1942 J. E. M. Thompson was instrumental in the beginning of the Instructional Course Lectures. During World War II, Major General Normal Kirk had established the concept of centralized treatment of regional diseases. With the war's end, the decentralization of the treatment centers was imminent, and in an effort to avoid complete loss of the teaching advantage inherent in the regional treatment of disease, the American Society for Surgery of the Hand was formed in 1945.

The evolution of the orthopedic publications took about as long as did the formation of the societies. With the formation of the AOA in 1887, the topics of discussion and papers presented at the meetings were published until 1903 as the Transactions of the AOA. In 1903 the Transactions ceased to exist and the first issue of the American Journal of Orthopedic Surgery was published. In 1918 when the publication became the official organ of the British Orthopedic Association as well, the name was again changed—this time to The Journal of Orthopedic Surgery. For reasons which are unclear, another change in name took place in 1922 with The Journal of Bone and Joint Surgery being the final choice. In 1935 the Journal of Bone and Joint Surgery became the official publication of the Academy as well.

This evolution of orthopedics hasn't been either a quick or an easy one. The development of the specialty had to wait, along with the other fields of medical endeavor, for hundreds of years while men learned enough about the basic social and physical sciences to provide a firm foundation on which medicine could build. It was some time after this before the men who had a special interest in diseases of the musculoskeletal system developed their knowledge and techniques to the point that they knew more about and were better able to handle the treatment of their special interest than were their contemporaries. It was only then that a man could say to his peers, "I am an orthopedic surgeon", and know that they knew that he was, and that he knew what he was talking about. The separation from general surgery hasn't been an easy job, but it was a necessary one, for according to Abel Phelps, "there never was a time when they could lie peacefully together in the same bed, excepting like the lion and the lamb—one inside the other, and the poor orthopedist was always inside".

Up to this point this monograph has dealt with the development of orthopedic surgery prior to the first half of the 20th century. The accomplishments of these great men became a springboard for an even more rapid advance in the treatment of maladies of bones and joints. I will mention some of the more important men and elaborate on their accomplishments in the list to follow.

CHAPTER 15
Newer advances in Orthopedic Surgery

Gerhard Küntscher performed what has now been called closed femoral rodding for femoral shaft fractures, by making a small incision above the level of the greater trochanter and inserting a cloverleaf-style rod in the medullary canal of the proximal segment, across the fracture site and on into the distal fragment thus stabilizing the femoral fracture. After the end of WWII U.S. Doctors were surprised to see American POWs returning from Germany soon after the fracture femur event with steel rods holding their fractures together. The next modification of placing transfixion screws into the intramedullary rod above and below the fracture site was brought into being by Grosse and Kempf who were under the impression that the distal screws should be removed after 6 weeks to allow "dynamizing" and prevent non-union. Doctors soon found that this 2nd procedure did not prove necessary in the majority of cases.

Another major event in the development of orthopedics in the 50s was the acceptance of arthroscopy. Masaki Watanabe of Japan had perfected the technique and instrumentation to the point where through a small incision pathology of the knee could be diagnosed and treated. Other joints soon came under the arthroscopic umbrella, and eventually minimal incision surgery became a goal in all cases.

In the early 1960s John Charnley of England had advanced his research on hip arthroplasty to the point where he was finding that polyethylene on metal gave the best interaction in the joint. By 1970 he published an article about his "low friction" arthroplasty that dramatically changed the outlook for those with hip arthritis and is no doubt one of the reasons why insurance tables now reveal that the average duration of life is approaching 80 since exercise upon a pain-free joint is more possible for many people.

Borge Walldius developed a hinge-joint type of replacement for the knee in 1951. Eventually the fully constrained replacement idea gave way to less constrained designs since the knee mechanics are such that there is too much force applied to components that are fixed in a one axial plane. The era of treatment of knee arthritis with a less constrained device was ushered in with the advent of the report in 1971 by Frank H. Gunston (of the Wrightington Hospital in Lancashire, England). He wrote of his experience with a low friction knee arthroplasty of a polycentric design. Since that time there has been concern about the many things that might go wrong—such as infection, loosening of components, phlebitis, and wear, but these problems have been ameliorated by proper selection of patients, the use of cemented components, anticoagulant measures, as well as the use of laminar air flow in the operating room. Certainly the results far outweigh the problems that previously existed with metal on metal components. Further improvements in design occurred with the constrained total knee of Coventry and still later the semi-constrained one of Insall and Burnstein. John Insall M.D. and Albert Burstein, a biomechanical engineer, developed their prosthesis at the Hospital for Special Surgery in Manhattan. Now there are four non-constrained knee choices: the UCI knee, Miller/Galante I or II and the Genesis of Richards Company. The majority of designs are manufactured by Zimmer and Howmedica, but there are about 10 other companies in this country and Europe making total knee components.

Hand deformity seen in rheumatoid arthritis became immeasurably improved after Alfred Swanson of Grand Rapids in 1962 developed silicone implants to replace destroyed and dislocated metatarso-phalangeal (knuckle) joints.

In the '60s Garriil Ilizarov of Russia perfected his technique of leg lengthening or shortening. In 1980 during the Cold War era Italian doctors became aware of his ability when a case of tibial nonunion was treated successfully by Ilizarov. The photojournalist involved had incurred the fracture 20 years before in a skiing accident.

Much progress has been made in spine surgery, and one of the most important contributors was Harold H. Bohlman, who was chief of the Acute Spinal Cord Injury Unit at the Veteran's Administration Medical Center and was Professor of Orthopedic Surgery and Director of the University Hospitals Spine Institute. He was President of the Cervical Spine Research Society in 1988-1989; President of the Federation of Spine Associations in 1994. He was Civilian National Consultant to the United States Surgeon General's Office for Spine Surgery. In 2006 he received the Leon T. Wiltse Award from the North American Spine Society. In 2008 he received the Nicolas Andry Award for Lifetime Achievement in Spine Surgery. He published 121 articles in peer review journals, 45 book chapters, and presented 445 lectures in the US and abroad. He was Director of the Spine Fellowship Program at the University Hospital Case Medical Center.

Another important spine surgeon was William Kirkaldy-Willis, who with Leon Wiltse, Harry Farfan, and Harry Crock founded the North American Spine Society. He was responsible for numerous publications including his four volume textbook "Managing Low Back Pain".

Leon T. Wiltse was an orthopedic surgeon at the Long Beach Memorial Hospital for over 50 years. He was a graduate of Northwestern University Feinberg School of Medicine in 1941. He had a special interest in spondylolisthesis and adhesive arachnoiditis secondary to the neurotoxicity of oil myelography.

He designed better implants and with Kirkaldy-Willis started the North American Spine Society. He became known as one of the great masters of low back surgery. He developed the Wiltse Spinal Fixation System in 1985.

During the 20th century there has been a large increase in the number of autos on the road as well as an increase in the number of DUIs and visits to the Emergency Room by those who partake in alcohol or drugs while driving or just falling asleep at the wheel.

In the past few decades there have been advances in the fields that aid the orthopedic surgeon accomplish his task better and improve patient care. For example, in radiology they not only have computer tomography (CT scans) but they also have the potential of obtaining 3D reconstruction and an MRI, both of which give a clearer picture of where internal fixation needs to be placed. This is especially true in fractures of the pelvis and dislocations of the sacro-iliac joint.

In the clinic and in the emergency room casts are applied for both acute and subacute fractures. In many cases fiberglass has taken the place of plaster. It came into being in the 70s and had to be cured (or hardened) using a "black light" for a few minutes. The development of fiberglass that could be activated by dipping the rolls in water advanced the use of fiberglass (which is lighter than plaster) to the point where almost all casts are applied with this material.

In the operating room it has become routine to have fluoroscopy available to direct the proper placement of plates and screws that hold the broken parts together. Not only that, but it is customary for the orthopedist to have small fluoroscopy units in the office as well as x-rays to diagnose the injury and amount of healing quicker.

In some cases a problem exists where there is either a lack of bone at the fracture site or the bone stops healing and becomes a non-union. To treat the lack of bone substance several allograft products have been developed: Dynagraft, Gafton, Opteform, Orthoblast, AlloMatrix, and Puros Allografts. In addition, there are commercially available bone substitute products as follows: Bioglass, Collagraft, Interpore, Norian Bone Paste, OsteoSet, and ProOsteon. Even further, there are substances called biochemical bone growth enhancers such as demineralized bone matrix, and bone morphogenic proteins.

Even the hardware used in fracture fixation has improved so that incompatible metals are not used together. Titanium alloys and stainless steel (composed of iron, chromium, and nickel) are the metals usually used. The need for compression at the fracture site was originally described by Key and later popularized by Charnley. Müller's group in Switzerland have designed a compression plate and equipment which have been upgraded several times since their introduction in 1963.

CHAPTER 16
Development of sub-specialties

Due to the complexity of the musculoskeletal system, there has been a tendency for orthopedic surgeons to specialize or concentrate their efforts in some aspect of the field that particularly interests them. Thus the Board of Specialty Societies (BOS) was created in 1984 to bring together the various leaders in each of the subspecialty disciplines in order to achieve excellence in each area. The BOS is now composed of 22 musculoskeletal specialty societies which are as follows:

1. American Association for Hand Surgery
2. American Association of Hip and Knee Surgeons.
3. American Orthopedic Foot and Ankle Society
4. American Orthopedic Society for Sports Medicine
5. American Shoulder and Elbow Surgeons
6. American Society for Surgery of the Hand
7. American Spinal Injury Association
8. Arthroscopy Association of North America
9. Cervical Spine Research Society
10. Hip Society
11. J. Robert Gladden Orthopaedic Society
12. Knee Society
13. Limb Lengthening and Reconstruction Society
14. Musculoskeletal Tumor Society
15. North American Spine Society
16. Orthopaedic Rehabilitation Association
17. Orthopaedic Research Society
18. Orthopaedic Trauma Association
19. Pediatric Orthopaedic Society of North America
20. Ruth Jackson Orthopaedic Society
21. Scoliosis Research Society

22. Society of Military Orthopaedic Surgeons

For the most part, membership in any of these societies requires that a candidate become certified by the ABOS. American Society for Surgery of the Hand also requires that a member hold a Certificate of Added Qualifications in Hand Surgery. As anyone can surmise, there is constant need to upgrade one's knowledge in any given field. Continuing medical education is the means by which the individual orthopedic surgeon can be updated in matters that concern his field of endeavor. At the week-long annual meeting held at different large cities in the early part of the year, new information can be acquired. A plethora of lectures and instructional courses and scientific exhibits requires one to prepare a schedule to determine which courses best fit his needs. In addition, various companies touting their products have their booths to try to convince one that their product is the best one made.

There is a national organization based in Illinois that is involved in furthering the scientific advances in the field. The Orthopedic Research and Educational Foundation (OREF) was founded in 1955 by the efforts of the American Orthopedic Association, the American Academy of Orthopaedic Surgery, and the Orthopedic Research Society. Since then they have raised over 100 million dollars. It is the only independent, surgeon-driven organization supporting research in the musculoskeletal area. Their mission is to raise funds to support research and education on diseases and injuries of bones, joints, nerves, and muscles.

There is plenty of opportunity for medical school graduates to improve the quality of life for those afflicted with diseases or injuries to their bodies. It is hoped that competent people will see the need to enter the specialty of orthopedic surgery and add to the history of orthopedics.

ADDENDUM

BRIEF DESCRIPTIONS OF IMPORTANT ORTHOPEDIC PERSONS

Abbott, Leroy C. (1890—1965) From 1930 to 1957 he was chief of the Department of Orthopedic Surgery at the University of California in San Francisco. He reported on his technique of leg lengthening in 1927.

Albee, Fred H. (1876—1945) New York orthopedist. AOA president 1929. Considered the "father of bone graft surgery". Became world famous for his treatment of spinal tuberculosis.

Albert, Eduard of Vienna. He stabilized a foot in 1878 and coined the term "arthrodesis". He was influential in establishing orthopedics as a specialty in Vienna.

Allis, Oscar H. (1836—1921) Philadelphia surgeon. Designed Allis clamp. First clinical Professor of Orthopedics at Jefferson Medical School. Work on etiology and prevention of spinal curvature.

Andry, Nicholas (1704—1756) French physician. Wrote "Orthopedia" at age 82 from which the term orthopedics was derived. Professor of Medicine at University of Paris.

Annandale, Thomas (1838—1907) Edinburgh surgeon. One of the earliest to do osteotomies for deformity. Known for his early work on meniscus injuries—1879.

Aufranc, Otto (1910—1990) Chairman of the orthopedic department in New England Baptist Hospital for 14 years starting in 1969. He was instrumental in developing the first replacement hip ("total hip arthroplasty") in the United States.

Axhausen, Georg (1877—1960) German pathologist. Monograph in 1908 on pathological anatomy of free bone transplants, in which he first described replacement of dead bone by living.

Baeyer, Hans von (1875—1941) Heidelberg. Professor of Orthopedics at Heidelberg until 1933. Worked on mechanics of muscular action and clinical kinetics. One of the earliest to suggest osteotomy.

Barlow, Thomas (1845—1945) English physician. Described the pathogenesis of infantile scurvy in 1882—Barlow's Disease.

Barton, John (1794—1871) Philadelphia. Professor of Surgery, University of Pennsylvania. Barton's fracture of the distal radius. Did the first femoral neck osteotomy in 1827 for an ankylosed hip.

Bauer, Louis (1814—1898) New York. Pupil of Stromeyer. Early American orthopedist who advocated Thomas principles in opposition to "American" method of "elastic traction".

Belchier, John (1706—1785) London. Did early experiments with madder staining the bone of living animals red. A London surgeon at Guy's Hospital.

Bell, Charles (1774—1842) Scottish physician. During early 1800s worked out and taught the functional anatomy of the central nervous system. Bell's palsy.

Bick, Edgar M. (1902—) New York. AOA member, associate editor of Clinical Orthopedics. Wrote "Source Book of Orthopaedics". Adjunct orthopedic surgeon, Hospital for Joint Diseases and Mount Sinai Hospital.

Biesalski, Konrad (1868—1930) German surgeon. Established the first rehab center in Europe—Oskar-Helene Heim. Did early experimental work on tendon surgery.

Bigelow, Henry J. (1818—1890) Boston. Published first account of Morton's ether anesthesia. Extensive writer on hip surgery. Described "Y" ligament of hip capsule. Professor of Surgery at Harvard.

Bircher, Eugen (1882—1956) Berne, Switzerland. Pioneer in the use of intramedullary control. Used ivory pegs in 1886. Introduced arthroscopy of the knee in 1921.

Bleck, Eugene E. (1923—) Palo Alto. Past President, American Orthopaedic Association, 1992. Past President, Pediatric Orthopaedic Society, 1983. Past President. American Academy for Cerebral Palsy and Developmental Medicine, 1976. Professor of Orthopaedic Surgery, Stanford University, and Chief, Pediatric Orthopaedic and Rehabilitative Services, Children's Hospital at Stanford, 1977. Professor and Chief of Division of Orthopaedic Surgery, Stanford University, 1982. Professor Emeritus, Orthopaedic Surgery, Stanford University, 1989—present. He has had 85 articles published in refereed journals and has authored three books on orthopaedic topics: 1) Atlas of Plaster of Paris Techniques, 1956, 2) Orthopaedic—Management of Cerebral Palsy, 1987. 3) Bleck, E.E. and Nagel, D. A. Physically Handicapped Children, a Medical Atlas for Teachers, 1975.

Blount, Walter (1900—1992) Milwaukee. Introduced epiphyseal stapling for growth abnormalities in the lower extremity. Wrote "Fractures in Children" and with John Moe wrote "The Milwaukee Brace".

Böhler, Thomas (1885—1973) Austrian surgeon. Had great influence on early treatment of fractures—early weight-bearing, unpadded casts, rehabilitation programs, blind intramedullary nailing.

Bohlman, Harold H. (1937—2010) Cleveland. Important contributor to spine surgery.

Borelli, Giovanni (1608—1679) Italian physiologist. Founder of theory of modern kinetics. Wrote "De Moto Animalium". A pupil of Galileo and teacher of Malphigi.

Brackett, E. G. (1860—1944) Boston. Brackett's operation for femoral neck fracture. Chief of Orthopedics at Massachusetts General Hospital and one time Director of Orthopedics, U.S. Army.

Bristow, Rowley (1882—1947) English orthopedist. Wrote estensively on repair of nerve and muscle injuries. Orthopedic surgeon to St. Thomas Hospital.

Brodie, Benjamin (1783—1862) England. Professor of Comparative Anatomy and Physiology at the Royal College of Surgeons in 1816. Gave lecture in 1845 on chronic abscess of tibia—now known as Brodie's abscess.

Bradford, E. H. (1848—1926) Boston. 3rd President of AOA. Professor of Orthopedic Surgery at Harvard in 1903. His Bradford table was originally used for treating congenital dislocation of the hip. He was active in preventive orthopedics.

Brown, Buckminster (1819—1891) Boston. Son of John Ball Brown, grandson of John Warren. In charge of the first orthopedic ward in New England at Samaritan Hospital, 1861. Had tuberculous spondylitis.

Buck, Gordon (1807—1877) New York. Buck's extension 1860 was initiated as traction treatment for femoral neck fracture. One of the founders of N. Y. Academy of Medicine. Wrote "Contributions to Reparative Surgery" in 1876.

Bunnell, Sterling (1882—1957) San Francisco. Laid the groundwork for the atraumatic technique of hand surgery.

Calot, François (1861—1944) French surgeon. Devised plaster jacket for correction of spinal deformity about 1895.

Campbell, Willis (1880—1941) Memphis. President AOA 1931 and Academy in 1934. First Professor of Orthopedics at Memphis. Did work with onlay bone graft, arthroplasty, paralytic deformities. In about 1935 he set down his knowledge in a text he called "Textbook of Orthopaedic Surgery". In 1939 Campbell's Operative Orthopaedics came into being, and is now considered the bible of orthopedic surgeons.

Camper, Peter (1722—1790) Dutch physician. Professor of Medicine at Amsterdam. Classic monograph on dynamic physiology of the foot in 1781.

Charcot, Jean M. (1825—1893) French neurologist. Described neurogenic arthropathy in 1868. Charcot-Marie-Tooth disease. Greatest neurologist of his day.

Charnley, John (1911—1982) Famous for his monograph "Compression Arthrodesis". He worked doggedly to improve the total hip joint arthroplasty resulting in what he termed "low friction arthroplasty" where polyethylene on metal worked much better than metal on metal. He also established the use of methylmethacrylate in stabilizing the femoral component. His article, "Arthroplasty of the Hip. A New Operation" was published in the Lancet in 1961.

Cheselden, William (1688—1752) English surgeon. Most outstanding surgeon of early 18th century. Wrote "Osteographia" in 1733. Dissected criminals in his home.

Chopart, Francis (1743—1795) French surgeon. Described disarticulation at the midtarsal level—now called Chopart's joint.

Chuliac, Guy de (1300—1368) Montpelier. Codified the accumulated writings of his time. The chief representative of medieval surgery. His "Chirurgia magna" introduced suspension and traction for fractures.

Codivilla, Alessandrio (1851—1913) Bologna. 2nd Director of the Rizzoli Institute. Did work on tendon transfer, stressing preservation of gliding mechanism.

Codman, Earnest A. (1869—1940) Boston. Founded the Registry of Bone Sarcoma in 1921 under the auspice of the American College of Surgeons. Codman's tumor, triangle.

Colles, Abraham (1773—1843) Dublin. Head of the Irish Royal College of Surgeons at age 29. "On Fracture of the Carpal Extremity of the Radius". "Treatise on Surgical Anatomy".

Cooper, Astley (1768—1841) English surgeon. Trained under John Hunter and became one of Europe's greatest teachers of surgery and anatomy.

Coventry, Mark (1913—1994) The brainchild for Mayo's unique tool for orthopedic research—the joint replacement database accumulated all the facts (since 1969) about the replacements on every knee, hip, shoulder, wrist, ankle, finger, and elbow done at the Mayo clinic. He was also known for high tibial osteotomy for treatment of osteoarthritis of the knee joint. He also did the first FDA approved total hip Arthroplasty. In 1973 he introduced the geometric prosthesis for knee arthritis—this had highly congruent (constrained) articular surfaces.

Cunningham, J. K. (1868—1932) Oklahoma city. Taught and promoted care of crippled children in southwest for 25 years.

Davis, Gwilyn G. (1857—1919) Philadelphia. Professor of Orthopedics, University of Pennsylvania. Developed surgical treatment for paralytic feet—his "Horizontal Transverse Section" operation. President of AOA in 1913.

Davis, H. G. (1807—1896) New York. The leading exponent of "elastic traction"—the American method of treatment in hip disease. Became a skilled bracemaker. One of the "big four" in early New York.

Delpech, J. M. (1777—1832) Montpelier, France. Pioneer orthopedic surgeon of France. Did first subcutaneous tenotomy in 1816—on an Achilles tendon.

Detmold, William (1808—1894) New York. Said to be New York's first orthopedic surgeon. First public clinic for treatment of crippled children. Brought Stromeyer's tenotomy to America.

Dillehunt, R. B. (1886—1953) Portland. First teacher of orthopedics in the northwest. Helped in the development of the Shriner's movement.

Duchenne, G. B. A. (1806—1875) French neurologist. "Des Movements" (1855)—a monograph on coordinated movement of the extremities. Wrote on muscle atrophies and dystrophies. Founder of electro-therapy.

Duhamel, Henri-Louis (1700—1782) Paris. Periosteal theory of oseogenesis. Showed madder to stain actively growing areas of bone only. Non-physician member of French Academy of Science.

Dunn, Naughton (1884—1939) Birmingham, England. Work on operative treatment of paralytic deformities of the foot. Trained with Jones at 11 Nelson Street.

Dupuytren, Guillaume (1777—1835) French surgeon. "On the Bones" (1846) Described contracture in palmar fascia in 1832. Endowed a museum.

Eikenbary, C. F. (1877—1933) Seattle. Influential in establishing the specialty of orthopedics in Seattle. A pupil of Ridlon and Whitman.

Elmslie, R. C. (1878—1940) London. In charge of Shepard's Bush Hospital during WWI. One of Great Britain's greatest teachers and philosophers of orthopedics.

Esmarch, Johann F. A. von (1823—1908) German surgeon. Devised the elastic rubber tourniquet as well as various operations including an amputation at the hip.

Fabrig, William (—) Performed a talectomy in 1608, which became the first published case

Fairbank, H. A. T. (1876—1961) England. Pupil of Lane. In charge of the first exclusively orthopedic service in England, at the Charing Cross Hospital in 1906. Wrote "Atlas of General Affections of the Skeleton".

Flatt, Adrian (1921—) Spent 22 years as a teacher at University of Iowa Medical Center He wrote nearly 200 publications and three books and was responsible for the development of a metal prosthesis for the rheumatoid hand (a steel hinge with two prongs) (the Flatt prosthesis) which was written up in a Time magazine article in December 1961 with the heading "Steel Knuckles". Among his many honors included being the past president of the American Society for Surgery of the Hand.

Freiberg, Albert H. (1868—1940) Cincinnati. AOA President 1911. First Professor of Orthopedics at University of Cincinnati. Called "The philosopher of orthopedics" by Leo Mayer.

Gallie, Willliam (1882—1959) Toronto. Did work on experimental bone grafting. Pioneer work on the use of free fascial grafts, tenodesis.

Gibney, Virgil P. (1847—1927) New York. First president of AOA and re-elected in 1912. Although no surgeon himself, he foresaw the operative future of orthopedics. He was Chief at Hospital for Ruptured and Crippled.

Girdlestone, Gathorne (1881—1950) In 1937 he became the first Nuffield Professor of Orthopedics. President of AOA in 1942. Did a hip resection for tuberculosis.

Gillette, Arthur (1864—1921) St. Paul. Instrumental in establishing the first state home for crippled children—in Minnesota. Professor of Orthopedics at Minnesota State University.

Glisson, Francis (1597—1677) English physician. A 400 plus page monograph dealing with rickets which was the first one in England dealing with a single disease.

Goldthwait, Joel (1866—1961) Boston. Chairman "Preparedness Committee" which went to work with Robert Jones at onset of WWI. Classic papers on sacro-iliac joint and posture. Preventive orthopedics.

Goodsir, John (1814—1867) Edinburgh. Demonstrated formation of bone by osteoblasts in 1852. Described the effect of "nuclear vascular membrane" (pannus) on cartilage.

Guerin, J. R. (1801—1886) French orthopedist who was supposed to have been the first to use a plaster bandage for splinting a corrected club foot. Did paravertebral myotomy for scoliosis.

Hall, Marshall (1790—1857) England. Established the concept of the reflex arc and the integrated function of muscles on a reflex basis.

Haller, Albrecht von (1708—1777) Swiss physiologist, anatomist, botanist. He backed the theory of arterial osteogenesis as opposed to Duhamel's theory of periosteal osteogenesis.

Harrington, Paul (1911—1980) Houston. Created apparatus for internal fixation and fusion of scoliosis both for polio victims as well as those afflicted with idiopathic scoliosis.

Havers, Clopton (1653—1702) English anatomist. First adequate description of bone and joint histology in "Osteologia Nova" around 1691. Described Haversian glands and canals.

Henry, Arnold K. (1886—1962) Dublin. Irish anatomist and surgeon who published "Extensile Exposure" in 1945 with a style unique among books on surgical approaches.

Hey, William (1736—1819) Leeds, England. Classic article on knee cartilages in 1803. Coined the term "internal derangement of the knee".

Hey Groves, Ernest W. (1872—1944) London. Did a cruciate repair in 1917 and inserted an ivory prosthesis in 1927. In bone grafting he established the priority of living grafts over autogenous, then homogenous, and finally heterogenous.

Hibbs, Russell (1869—1932) New York. Replaced Shaffer at New York Orthopedic Dispensary. Announced his spine fusion operation almost simultaneously with Albee.

Hilton, John (1804—1878) English surgeon and anatomist. Established the principle of rest in "On Rest and Pain" in 1863. Hilton's Law: In a given joint the muscles that move it and the skin over it have a common innervation.

Hoffa, Albert (1859—1911) German orthopedist. Developed an open reduction for CDH in 1890. Active surgeon who did early operative work on many problems in orthopedics.

Hoffman, Phillip (1870—1939) St. Louis. Resection of metatarsal heads as treatment for claw toes.

Hoke, Michael (1874—1944) Atlanta. AOA 1926. Enlisted support of Shriners in care of crippled children. F.D.R.'s orthopedist. Famous for work on club feet.

Hunt, Dame Agnes (1867—1948) Liverpool. Established the basic pattern of the central hospital with after-care clinics in England. Jones called her "the Florence Nightingale of orthopedic nursing".

Hunter, John (1728—1793) Scottish surgeon. Established scientific basis for surgery with his studies in anatomy, physiology, and experimental pathology. The Hunterian Museum of Royal College of Surgeons was named after him.

Hunter, William (1718—1783) England. John's brother. Did basic work on the nutrition of articular cartilage. Described arteriovenous aneurysm.

Ilizarov, Gavriil A. (1921—1992) Soviet physician who practiced in Siberia. In 1961 he created the Kurgan Center of the Restorational Surgery and Orthopedy. He is famous for advancing the operation of leg lengthening started by Leroy C. Abbott, Harold Sofield and M. V. Anderson by performing distraction osteogenesis using his Ilizarov apparatus—this was described in a 1971 article.

Insall, John (1930—2000) New York. English-trained orthopedic surgeon, who designed four models of widely used systems for total knee replacement. In 1976 introduced the first tricompartment total knee arthroplasty—the unconstrained total condylar knee replacement.

Jansen, Mürk (1867—1935) Leyden. Dutch surgeon who brought the British and American pattern of orthopedics to Holland, displacing the old German methods. Established the Anna Kliniek and wrote "On Bone Formation" in 1920.

Jones, Robert (1858—1911) Liverpool. Established orthopedics as a specialty in England. Nephew of H. O. Thomas, whose principles he helped to establish. Was involved in tendon transfer, bone grafting, and rehabilitation.

Jones, S. Fosdick (1874—1946) Denver. Pennsylvanian who became a pupil of Gibney. After coming to Denver in 1906, he became Professor of Orthopedic Surgery at the University of Colorado Medical School. He had tuberculosis.

Judson, A. B. (1837—1916) New York. President of AOA in 1891. Outstanding for his work on scoliosis in which he demonstrated the rotary element.

Kanavel, Allen B. (1874—1938) American surgeon. Contributed greatly to the surgical and pathological anatomy of infections of the hand which he described in his book in 1939.

Keith, Arthur (1866—1955) Scottish anthropologist, anatomist. Wrote "Menders of the Maimed" in 1919. With Flack he discovered the sino-atrial node.

Key, J. Albert (1890—1955) St. Louis. Instituted compression arthrodesis of the knee for tuberculosis in 1932.

Kirkaldy-Willis, William (1914—2006) Saskatoon, Canada. A primary founder of the North American Spine Society.

Kirmisson, Edouard (1848—1927) French surgeon who directed the development of orthopedic surgery in early France. Organized and became first president of French Orthopedic Society.

Kleinberg, Samuel (1886—1957) America orthopedist who wrote extensively on scoliosis, spondylolisthesis, and CDH. Devised operation for internal rotation contracture of the shoulder.

Knight, James (1810—1877) New York. Founder of Hospital for Ruptured and Crippled in 1863. An extreme conservative who used braces and did no surgery. The Knight back brace was named after him. He was one of the original "big four".

Koch, Robert (1843—1901) German bacteriologist. Discovered tubercle bacillus in 1882. Introduced tuberculin vaccine in 1890. He was one of the founders of modern bacteriology.

Kocher, Emil T. (1841—1917) Swiss surgeon. Kocher's method of shoulder reduction. Devised operations for excision of hip and ankle. Nobel laureate in 1909. Kocher's forceps.

Küntscher, Gerhard (1900—1972) German surgeon. His first intramedullary nail was inserted in 1939. He performed several more procedures between 1942 and 1944 in the Finnish Lapland. The German military allowed it to be performed starting in 1942 and by the end of the war returning POWs revealed the evidence of steel (Küntscher) rods in their femurs with small incisions on the ipsilateral buttocks. A. W. Fischer in 1944 considered the Küntscher nailing a great revolution.

Lambotte, Albin (1866—1955) Antwerp, Belgium. Contemporary of Lane who developed methods of internal fixation of fractures around 1900. Used screw-plate fixation.

Lane, Arbuthnot (1856—1943) London. Scottish surgeon famous for his "no touch" technique. Established the principles of internal fixation in his "Operative Treatment of Fractures" in 1905.

Lange, Fritz (1864—1952) Munich. Did work on tendon transfer. He worked out a method of subperiosteal implantation and was one of the earliest to attempt to fuse the spine.

Langenbeck, Bernhard R. K. von (1810—1887) German surgeon from Berlin. Did the first subcutaneous osteotomy around 1882. In 1850 he treated a femoral neck fracture by placing a screw through the greater trochanter into the head.

Leriche, Rene (1879—1955) Lyon, France. French surgeon who did pioneer work in vascular/peripheral nerve surgery and described in 1940 the use of sympathectomy to increase peripheral blood supply. He did original work on physiology and pathology of bone. Leriche syndrome = impotence and buttock claudication. In 1924 he was appointed Professor of Surgery at the University of Strassbourg and was the first surgeon to become Professor at the College of France.

Leveuf, Jacques (1886—1948) French surgeon. Wrote extensively on Volkmann's contracture, osteomyelitis, and CDH for which he advocated open reduction.

Lister, Joseph (1827—1912) Edinburgh. Established the antiseptic method of surgey. Professor of Surgery at the

University of Edinburgh, replacing Syme, whose daughter he married. Active in the field of preventive medicine.

Little, E. Muirhead (1854—1935) London. Son of William John. First president of BOA. Wrote "Artificial Limbs and Amputation Stumps".

Little, William J. (1810—1894) English surgeon. Popularized technique of heel cord tenotomy. A patient and pupil of Stromeyer. Established the Orthopedic Institute of London.

Lorenz, Adolf (1854—1946) Austrian surgeon. He received the nickname "The Bloodless Surgeon of Vienna" for his non-invasive techniques, especially in treatment of CDH and clubfoot deformity.

Lucas-Championnierre, Just (1843—1913) French physician who was an unyielding advocate of movement in treatment of fractures. Taught that movement and massage at the fracture site were curative.

Macewen, William (1845—1924) Scottish surgeon. Performed the first premeditated homologous bone graft. Invented the osteotome. Wrote a monograph in 1912 on "The Growth of Bone". Greatest Scottish surgeon of his time.

Malgaigne, Joseph F. (1806—1865) French surgeon. Introduced skeletal fixation in 1847. Malgaigne's amputation (subtalar disarticulation). Malgaigne's fracture of the pelvis.

Mathijsen, Antonius (1805—1878) Flemish Army surgeon who initiated the use of Plaster of Paris (impregnated mesh bandage) in 1852 as a substitute for braces in deformity and fractures.

Mayer, Leo (1884—1972) New York orthopedist who worked with Lange and later Biesalski. Wrote extensively on the physiology of tendon transfer.

McMurray, Thomas P. (1888—1940) Liverpool. In 1938 he became the first Professor of Orthopedics at the University of Liverpool. Also in 1938 he described upper femoral osteotomy for osteoarthritis of the hip.

Minnius, Isacius (—) Dutch surgeon. Performed the first tenotomy for wryneck in 1685. The originator of subcutaneous tenotomy.

Moore, Austin T. (1889—1963) Columbia, South Carolina. With Harold Bohlman in 1942 reported the use of a metal prosthesis to replace a giant cell tumor of the proximal end of the femur. Later popularized his prosthesis for fractures of the femoral neck.

Moore, James E. (1852—1918) A leading Chicago orthopedist prior to 1900. Professor of Orthopedics at University of Minnesota in 1908. Author of text, "Orthopedic Surgery", published in 1898.

Morris, Sir William (Lord Nuffield) (—) Gave 125,000 pounds in the cause of Britain's cripples. Nuffield Professorship established at Oxford. His friendship with Girdlestone resulted in the first endowed chair of orthopedics in Britain.

Morton, Thomas G. (1835—1903) Philadelphia. One of the founders of Philadelphia Orthopedic Hospital in 1867. Described metatarsalgia in 1875. First successful laparotomy for appendicitis in 1886.

Mott, Valentine (1785—1865) New York. First to use term "orthopedic surgery". Prominent as a vascular surgeon and did a lot of orthopedic operations gaining prestige for that specialty.

Murphy, John B. (1857—1916) American surgeon. Developed the fascia-fat membrane arthroplasty about 1904 and introduced it in this country. Responsible for the Murphy sign in perinephritic abscess.

Nelaton, Aguste (1807—1873) French surgeon. In 1847 described the line which immediately became the popular measure for clinical diagnosis of CDH. Also, described numerous orthopedic operations.

Nesbitt, Robert (1700—1761) Wrote "Human Osteogeny" in 1731. He gave a good description of endochondral and intramembranous bone formation.

Nichols, Edward H. (1864—1922) Boston. First good pathological description of tuberculosis of bone and joint. An able surgeon who was also Associate Professor in Surgical Pathology.

Nicola, Toufick (1894—) American orthopedist most widely known for his biceps transfer repair of recurrent dislocation of the shoulder.

Nicoladoni, Karl (1847—1902) Austrian surgeon who reintroduced tendon transfer, using peroneal tendons into the Achilles tendon for paralytic equinus deformity in 1882.

Ober, Frank (1861—1925) American orthopedist who devised a number of operations designed to alleviate paralysis. Ober's test for tight ilio-tibial band was named after him.

Ollier, Louis X. (1830—1900) French surgeon. Described multiple exostoses in 1898. Gave the clearest concept of bone growth and repair of his time. Experimented in bone grafting around 1859.

Orr, Winnett (1877—1956) Lincoln, Nebraska. Chief surgeon at Nebraska Orthopedic Hospital. Orthopedic historian and originator of Orr method of treatment for osteomyelitis.

Osgood, Robert (1873—1956) Boston. Described oseochondritis of the tibial tubercle in 1903. (He thought it was an avulsion.) He developed the popliteal approach to knee joint.

Packard, George B. (1852—1928) Denver. Founded department of orthopedics and Grosse Medical College, where he was Professor until 1919. President of the AOA in 1915. Early associate of Gibney and Shaffer.

Paget, James (1814—1899) English surgeon. Described osteitis deformans in 1876—now called Paget's disease.

Paracelsus (aureoles Philipus Theophrastus Bombastus ab Hohenheim) (1493—1541) Swiss physician. Began the use of chemical agents alone as treatment of disease. Father of chemotherapy.

Paré, Ambrose (1510—1590) French surgeon and pioneer bracemaker. Applied ligature to amputation instead of hot oil. Greatest surgeon of his time and considered the father of modern medicine.

Park, Roswell (1852—1914) Buffalo. Wrote "Epitome of the History of Medicine". A teacher of orthopedic surgery and was Professor of Surgery at the University of Buffalo in 1883.

Parker, Rushton (1848—1932) Liverpool, England. Professor of Surgery at the University of Liverpool. He was successful in getting H. O. Thomas to get his ideas and experience into print.

Pasteur, Louis (1822—1951) French bacteriologist. Proved that putrefaction was the result of bacteria, rather than "spontaneous generation". Founded Pasteur Institute in Paris.

Payr, Erwin (1871—1947) German surgeon. In 1913 he attempted to substitute trapezius motor for paralyzed deltoid. He also published work on arthroplasty.

Phelps, Winthrop M. (1894—1971) Baltimore. In 1931 he became chief of orthopedic surgery at the Yale University School of Medicine. In 1936 he moved to Baltimore and established the Children's Rehabilitation Institute. His publication in 1932 giving the classification of cerebral palsy was considered a significant contribution by Edgar M. Bick.

Phelps, Abel M. (1851—1902) New York. Professor of Orthopedics at Vermont; later he founded the Department of Orthopedics at New York Postgraduate Medical School and Hospital in 1887. He devised several clubfoot operations and was an enemy of the proponents of "strap and buckle" usage.

Phemister, D. B. (1882—1951) Chicago. Outstanding researcher and teacher in bone and joint pathology. Described graft techniques, epiphyseal arrest.

Physick, Phillip Syng (1768—1837) Philadelphia. First Professor of Surgery at the University of Pennsylvania. First to use absorbable suture in this country. An outstanding surgeon who had an interest in orthopedics.

Platt, Sir Harry (1886—1986) Emeritus Professor of Orthopedic Surgery in the University of Manchester. He was in charge of the first fracture service in England at Ancoats Hospital in Manchester. His name endures in the Putti-Platt type of shoulder procedure for recurrent dislocation.

Pott, Percival (1714—1788) English surgeon. Described the deformity and sequellae of spinal tuberculosis, but not its tuberculous nature. Pott's ankle fracture. Essay on "Fractures and Dislocations".

Putti, Vittorio (1880—1940) Bologna. 3rd director of the Rizzoli Institute. He did a great deal of work on the treatment and prevention of CDH.

Recklinghausen, F. D. von (1833—1910) German pathologist. Described osteitis fibrosa cystic in 1892. This became known as von Recklinghausen's neurofibromatosis.

Redfern, Peter (1821—1912) Aberdeen. English anatomist/ physiologist. Did basic research in the physiology of cartilage—its method of repair and reaction to injury.

Ridlon, John (1852—1936) Chicago. Professor of Orthopedics, Northwestern in 1890. Taught techniques of H. O. Thomas and Robert Jones in America. He was politically powerful in AOA activities from late 1800s to early 1900.

Rizzoli, Francesco (1809—1880) Bologna. Italian surgeon who endowed the Rizzoli Institute at Bologna in 1880, and it became a mecca for young orthopedic surgeons from all over the world.

Roentgen, William (1845—1923) German physicist. X-rays discovered in 1894. Nobel laureate in 1901.

Rusk, Howard (1901—1989) First Professor of Rehabilitation in the United States. He was the founder of the Rusk Institute of Rehabilitative Medicine.

Ryerson, E. W. (1872—1961) Chicago. First president of American Academy of Orthopedic Surgeons. He devised an anterior talar bone block operation for paralytic pes calcaneous.

Salter, Robert B. (1924—2010) Toronto. He developed the concept of continuous passive motion which is used in a wide variety of orthopedic conditions. He created the "Salter operation" for treating CDH. He established the first clinical fellowship program in orthopedics in North America. In 1957 he became chief of orthopedic surgery at the Hospital for Sick Children in Toronto.

Sayre, Louis (1820—1900) New York. First Professor of Orthopedics in the United States—at Bellevue Hospital in 1861. In 1854 he did the first successful hip joint resection. He was elected to the AOA two years after his son Reginald was elected.

Sayre, Reginald (1859—1929) New York. Club hand operation in 1893. An advocate of preventive orthopedics. He became a president of the AOA.

Schede, Max (1844—1902) Bonn. He was supposedly the first to discover the role of anteversion in redislocation of a treated CDH in 1897. In 1900 he published a monograph on CDH.

Scudder, Charles L. (1860—1949) Boston. Established the first complete fracture service at Massachusetts General Hospital. He wrote "Treatment of Fractures" which has gone through 11 editions.

Sever, James (1878—1964) Boston. Sever's disease is epiphysitis of the os calcis. Known for Sever's operation to release an internal rotation contracture of the shoulder. He became head of the department at the Boston City Hospital.

Shaffer, Newton M. (1846—1928) New York. An organizer of AOA and 2nd president. He was a surgeon-in-chief at the New York Orthopedic Dispensary. Quoted as saying, "To mingle surgery and mechanics is to endanger both".

Shanz, Alfred (1870—1932) Dresden. German surgeon who had an extensive knowledge of braces and appliances. He developed his "abduction osteo-osteotomy". He wrote a textbook on orthopedics in 1908.

Sherman, Harry (1854—1921) San Francisco. Clinical Professor of Orthopedics at the University of California. President of the AOA in 1900. He was the first orthopedist in California.

Smith-Peterson, Marius N. (1886—1953) Boston. Famous for his work on anatomy ad pathology of the hip, as well as his arthroplasty and treatment of femoral neck fractures.

Sprengel, Otto G. K. (1852—1915) German surgeon. He was the first to use an ilio-femoral incision and his eponym appears on the deformity of a scapula that fails to descend during fetal life. Although he described it in 1891, Albert Eulenberg had previously done the same in 1863.

Starr, Clarence (1867—1920) Canadian surgeon who worked at the Hospital for Sick Children. Founder of Canadian orthopedics.

Steele, A. J. (1835—1917) St. Louis. Professor of Orthopedics at Washington University. President of the AOA in 1893.

Steindler, Arthur (1828—1957) Born in Vienna. Professor of Orthopedics at Iowa University from 1913 to 1949. He was one of orthopedics' greatest teachers and surgeons and a prolific writer in the field. He described many operations.

Steinmann, N. Fritz (1872—1932) Bern, Switzerland. In 1907 he instituted skeletal traction by using his eponymic nail or pin, driving through the distal femur (and attaching suitable weights via a wire) to treat a fractured femur. This proved much more effective than skin traction and was considered one of the half dozen important contributions to fracture therapy in over 200 years of practice. Although Martin Kirschner introduced his smaller wire two years later, the Steinmann pin is still in vogue for effective traction.

Stoffel, Adolf (1880—1927) Mannheim. German surgeon. Devised the operation of neurectomy for spastic paralysis.

Stromeyer, George F. L. (1804—1876) Hanover. German surgeon who divided W. J. Little's contracted hell cord. One of the earliest to practice subcutaneous tenotomy.

Swanson, Alfred (1923—) Director emeritus of the Grand Rapids Orthopedic Surgery Program (Retired in June 2001) In 1962 he developed the one-piece silicone implant which revolutionized the treatment of the rheumatoid hand and proved more durable than previous metallic implants.

Taylor, C. F. (1827—1899) New York. Organized New York Orthopedic Dispensary in 1866. Developed his "spinal assistant" to prevent deformity in tuberculous spondylitis.

Thomas, Hugh O. (1834—1891) Liverpool. First physiologically and scientifically oriented orthopedic surgeon. Classic monograph on "Diseases of the Hip, Knee and Shoulder", available in 1962 reprint.

Tubby, A. H. (1863—1930) Westminster. "Orthopedic surgery is the surgery of the entire locomotor apparatus". His book, "Deformities: a Treatise on Orthopedic Surgery", was internationally read. Told the world in 1912 what he thought orthopedics should entail.

Velpeau, Alfred A. L. M. (1795—1867) French surgeon who called the deformity in Colles' fracture a "silver fork" deformity. Devised the "Velpeau bandage" still in use today.

Venel, Jean A. (1740—1791) Geneva physician. Established the Institute for Skeletal Deformities at Orbe, Switzerland in 1790—the first of its kind in the world.

Vesalius, Andreas (1514—1564) Flemish anatomist—probably the greatest anatomist of all time. "De humani corporis fabrica" was his classical book on anatomy.

Volkmann, Richard von (1830—1889(German surgeon. Discovered the carcinogenic effect of coal tar. Describe Volkmann's contracture—a serious deformity following poorly treated fractures above the elbow.

Vulpius, Oscar (1867—1936) Heidelberg. An early exponent of tendon transfer. Had a special interest in deformities caused by poliomyelitis.

Watanabe, Masaki (1921—1994) He was a student of Kenji Takagi who in 1918 had performed arthoscopy on a cadaver knee. During the 50s he was able to advance the technology of arthroscopes, and by 1957 published with his colleagues an "Atlas of Arthroscopy". Arthroscopy is now considered one of the biggest orthopedic advancements and is used for most of the major joints. It is not only used for diagnosis but also for repair and reconstruction. Robert W. Jackson, a Canadian orthopedic surgeon, in 1964 went to Japan and in the process of teaching Dr. Watanabe English learned about his use of arthroscopy. He then performed the first knee arthroscopy in 1967 in North America. With the help of advances in fiber optics in the 70s and 80s arthroscopy has become ubiquitous. In the states Richard L. O'Connor (1933—1980) made contributions both in the development of instruments and techniques, but also in the training of his colleagues in the methods of arthroscopy. At least 6 other doctors from countries like Italy, Germany, Switzerland and Denmark had made contributions to the development of arthroscopy starting in the early 1800s.

Watkins, James T. (1871—1934) San Francisco. Original member AOA. He formed the Pacific Coast Orthopedic Association, and was one of the chief figures in establishment of the Western Orthopedic Association. He was an associate of Harry Sherman.

Watson-Jones, Sir Reginald (1902—1972) He was a gifted surgeon, writer, educator and editor. He wrote "Fractures and Joint Injuries" which was published in 1940 and reprinted 15 times. He was the first editor of the British volume of the Journal of Bone and Joint Surgery.

Whitman, Royal (1857—1946) New York. One of the outstanding scholars of orthopedics. A brilliant and prolific writer and teacher. Known for Whitman's talectomy.

Willard, DeForest (1846—1910) Philadelphia. Professor of Orthopedics, University of Pennsylvania Medical School. 4th President of AOA. Established the first ward for crippled children at the University of Pennsylvania; also organized the first Social Service Department.

Wilson, Harry A. (1853—1919) Philadelphia. 2nd Professor of Orthopedics at Jefferson. First orthopedist to attend Philadelphia General Hospital. He introduced soluble compressed hypodermic tablets in 1885.

Wiltse, Leon F. (1913—2005) One of the founders of the North American Spine Society which is responsible for giving his eponymic award annually for excellence in spine surgery.

Wolff, Julius (1836—1923) Berlin. German surgeon and anatomist. Studied architectural morphology of bone. Wolff's Law (see page 18) promulgated in 1884.

BIBLIOGRAPHY

Adamson, J. E. J. Bone & Joint Surg., 43-A:709-716, 1961. History of flexor tendon grafting.

Albee, Fred H. Hygea 5:129-130; 131-134, 1927. 25 years with the orthopedic surgeon.

Albee, Fred H. W. B. Saunders, 1915. Bone Graft Surgery.

Bauer, Louis Lindsay & Blakiston. Philadelphia, 1864. Lectures on Orthopedic Surgery.

Bick, Edgar M. Williams & Wilkins, 1937. Source Book of Orthopedics.

Bick, Edgar M. J. B. Lippincott Co., 1976 Classics of Orthopaedics.

Bowman, A. K. J. Bone & Joint Surg., 26:495-502, 1944.

Brailsford, J. F. J. Int. Coll. Surg., 35:119-133, 1961. A Briton's contributions to Orthopedic Surgery.

Brockbank, William J. Bone & Joint Surg, 32-B:274-8, 1950. Luxations of the hip—16th and 17th centuries.

Brockbank, William J. Bone & Joint Surg., 30-B:365-75, 1948. Luxations of the shoulder—16th & 17th centuries.

Brockbank, William J. Bone & Joint Surg., 30-B:556-9, 1948. Luxations of the spine—16th & 17th centuries.

Brockbank, William J. Bone & Joint Surg., 30-B:714-22, 1948. The art of osteography.

Brockbank, William J Bone & Joint Surg., 31-B:472-5, 1949. Dismembering—16th & 17th centuries.

Brown, Buckminster David Clapp & Son, Boston, 1868. Cases in Orthopedic Surgery.

Buxton, J. D. J Bone & Joint Surg., 38-B4-21, 1956. Sir Thomas Fairbank.

Carr, E. F. Quart Bull N-W Med Sch. 20:441-7, 1946. Early medical books in Archibald Church library.

Carruthers, F. W. South Med J. 34:1223-26, 1941. Review of metals used in orthopedics.

Chatterton, Carl C. Minn. Med., 36: 360-3, 1953. Early orthopedic surgery in Minnesota.

Clendening, Logan Dover Publications, Inc., New York, 1942. Source book of medical history.

Cleveland, Mather J Bone & Joint Surg., 39-A:661-8, 1957. Traction versus rest in treatment of hip disease.

Cleveland, Mather Instruct. Course Lect., Am Acad of Ortho Surg., V-2: 228-39, 1948. Orthopedic Surgeons of the 19th century, New York.

Coates, Milsom J Bone & Joint Surg., 32-B: 611-14, 1950. First half-century of orthopedics in New Zealand.

Deyerle, W. N Eng J Med., 266:820-2, 1962. 100 year follow-up in case of internal fixation.

Dobson, Jessie J Bone & Joint Surg., 34-B: 702-7, 1952. Clopton Havers.

Dobson, Jessie J Bone & Joint Surg., 30-B: 551-5, 1948. Robert Nesbitt on human osteogeny.

Edelstein, J. M. J Bone & Joint Surg., 32-B: 615-17, 1950. Development of orthopedic surgery in south Africa.

Freiberg, Joseph A. J Bone & Joint Surg., 44-A: 1699-1702, 1962. Reflections on Orthopedic Surgery.

Girdlestone, G. R. J Bone & Joint Surg., 30-B: 189-95, 1948. The Robert Jones tradition.

Goldthwait, J. L. J. B. Lippincott Co., 1934. Body Mechanics in the Study and Treatment of Disease.

Green, William H. J Bone & Joint Surg., 39-A: 675-85, 1957. Orthopedic surgery, today, yesterday, and tomorrow.

Griffiths, D. L. J Bone & Joint Surg., 32-B: 676-93, 1950. Some classics of British orthopedic Literature.

Griffiths, D. L. J bone & Joint Surg., 31-B: 313-17, 1949. Traction apparatus…16th & 17th centuries.

Hall, Courtney Bull Hist. Med., 26: 231-62, 1952. Rise of professional surgery in the United States.

Harris, R. I. J Bone & Joint Surg., 32-B: 587-600, 1950. 50 years of orthopedic surgery in Canada.

Jackson, G. H. Arch. Surg., 46: 666-72, 1943. Henry Jacob Bigelow.

Jeffery, C. C. J Bone & Joint Surg., 41-B: 368-9, 1959. A fracture plated by W. A. Lane in 1912.

Jones, A. R. J Bone & Joint Surg., 38-B: 27-45, 1956. Review of orthopedic surgery in Great Britain.

Jones, A. R. J Bone & Joint Surg., 32-B: 126-30, 1950. Abraham Colles.

Jones A. R. J Bone & Joint Surg., 32-B: 425-8, 1950. Francis Glisson.

Jones, A.R. J Bone & Joint Surg., 35-B: 309-19, 1953. Influence of H. O. Thomas on treatment of skeletal tuberculosis.

Jones, A. R. J Bone & Joint Surg., 35-B: 661-6, 1953. John Haddy James.

Jones, A. R. J Bone & Joint Surg., 34-B: 123-8, 1952. Sir William Macewen.

Jones, A. R. J bone & Joint Surg., 34-B: 478-82, 1952. Sir William Arbuthnot Lane.

Jones, A. R. J Bone & Joint Surg., 36-B: 496-01, 1954. B. C. Brodie.

Jones, A. R. J Bone & Joint Surg., 35-B: 139-43, 1953. Alfred Herbert Tubby.

Jones, A. R. J Bone & Joint Surg., 33-B: 124-9, 1951. William Adams.

Jones, A. R. J Bone & Joint Surg., 31-B: 123-6, 1949. William John Little.

Jones, A. R. Proc.: R. Soc. Med., 31: 19-26, 1937. Evolution of orthopedics in Great Britain.

Jones, A. R. J Bone & Joint Surg., 30-B: 196-200, 1948. Joseph Lister.

Jones, A. R. J Bone & Joint Surg., 30-B: 357-60, 1948. John Hunter.

Jones, A. R. J Bone & Joint Surg., 30-B: 547-50, 1948. Hugh Owen Thomas.

Jones, A. R. J Bone & Joint Surg., 31-B: 465-70, 1949. Percival Pott.

Jones, Robert Oxford University Press, 1921. Orthopedic Surgery of Injuries.

Joy, Robert Bull Hist. Med., 28: 416-41, 1954. The natural bonesetters...the Sweet family.

Keith, Arthur Oxford University Press, 1919. Menders of the Maimed.

Kelley and Burrage D. Appleton & Co., New York, 1928. Dictionary of American Medical Biography.

Knight, James J. H. Vail & Co., 1884. Orthopaedia.

Lane, W. A. Lancet, 2: 1500-01, 1893. On the advantages of the steel screw in fracture treatment.

Lewin, Phillip Inst. Course Lect., Am Acad. Ortho Surg., V-2: 244-8, 1948. John Ridlon.

Luck, J. V. J Bone & Joint Surg., 44-A: 390-7, 1962. Orthopedic surgery...shaping it for permanence or ending.

Marti-Ibanez, F. M. D. Publications, Inc., New York, 1959. History of American Medicine...a symposium.

Mayer, Leo J Bone & Joint Surg., 37-A: 374-383, 1955. Reflections on some interesting personalities in orthopedic surgery.

Mayer, Leo J Bone & Joint Surg., 32-B: 461-569, 1950. Development of orthopedic surgery in the United States.

Miller, G. Bull Hist. Med., 36: 535-70, 1962. Bibliography of United States medical history.

Müller, M. E., Algöwer, M., Schneider, R., and Willenegger, H: Manual of internal fixation: techniques recommended by the AO/ASIF group, ed. 3, Berlin, 1990, Springer-Verlag.

Nicholson, J. T. Inst. Course Lect., Am Acad. Ortho. Surg., V-2: 239-44, 1948. 19th century orthopedics in Philadelphia.

Orr, H. Winnett Thomas, 1949. On the contributions of H. O. Thomas, R. Jones, and J. Ridlon.

Orr, H. Winnett Inst Course Lecture, Am Acad. Ortho Surg., V-10: 417-422, 1953. Motion and rest in bone and joint disease.

Orr, H. Winnett Inst Course Lect., Am Acad. Ortho Surg., V-10: 423-8, 1953. The operative treatment of non-union in fractures.

Orr, H. Winnett Inst Course Lect., Am Acad. Ortho Surg., V-2: 225-38, 1948. History of orthopedic surgery in western United States before 1900.

Orr, H. Winnett Inst Course Lect., Am Acad. Ortho Surg., V-9: 423-47, 1952. History and biography of orthopedic surgery.

Orr, H. Winnett Inst Course Lect., Am Acad. Ortho Surg., V-13: 307-19, 1956. Medical education and the orthopedic specialty in America.

Osgood, Robert D. C. V. Mosby Co., St. Louis, 1925. The evolution of orthopedic surgery.

Osmond-Clarke, H. J Bone & Joint Surg., 32-B: 620-75, 1950. Half a century of orthopedic progress in Great Britain.

Peltier, L. F. Surg. Gyn. Ob., 114: 252-5, 1962. Bonesetting.

Peltier, L. F. Norman Publishing. San Francisco, 1993. Orthopedics—A History and Iconography.

Platt, Harry J Bone & Joint Surg., 32-B: 570-86, 1950. Orthopedics on continental Europe, 1900-1950.

Podalsky, E. Am. J Surg., 74: 109-11, 1947. Four pioneers in bone: Knight, Taylor, Sayre, Davis.

Price, G. Quart Bull N-W Med Sch., 20: 449-63, 1946. History of surgical anesthesia.

Putti, Vittorio Hoebey, 1930. Historic artificial limbs.

Robertson, J. H. G. J Bone & Joint Surg., 32-B: 618-19, 1950. Orthopedic surgery in southern Rhodesia.

Robinson, Victor Froben Press, New York, 1938. Syllabus of medical history.

R. S. L.—In Memorium J Bone & Joint Surg., 38-B: 576-7, 1956. Lambotte, Albin—in memorium.

Sayre, Louis A. D. Appleton & Co., 1883. Lectures on Orthopedic Surgery and Diseases of Joints.

Shands, A. R. Jr. Clin. Ortho., 23: 1-10, 1962. Biography of Albee.

Stanisvljevic, S. Henry Ford Hosp Bull., 10: 257-61, 1962. Vittorio Putti and Willis C. Campbell.

Sofield, H. A. J Bone & Joint Surg., 42-A: 344-349, 1960. Growth of the vineyards.

Thomas, H. O. Little, Brown & Co., 1962 (1876). Diseases of the hip, knee and ankle joints.

Thompsen, W. E. J Bone & Joint Surg., 35-B: 298-308, 1953. Orthopedic Instruments.

Watson-Jones, R. J Bone & Joint Surg., 32-B: 694-729, 1950. Medullary nailing of fractures after 50 years.

Watson-Jones, R. J Bone & Joint Surg., 30-B: 709-13, 1948. Dame Agnes Hunt.

White, J. W. J Bone & Joint Surg., 37-A: 1101-9, 1958. Development of orthopedic surgery in the far west.

Whitman, Royal J Bone & Joint Surg., 26: 331-42, 1934. Critical estimate of the influence of Knight, Sayre, Thomas.

Whitman, Royal J Bone & Joint Surg., 16: 331-42, 1934. Critical estimate of Personal influence of four pioneers.

Whitman, Royal J Bone & Joint Surg., 29: 250-53, 1947. Evolution of orthopedics in New York City.

Whitman, Royal Am J Surg., 41: 129-32, 1938. American orthopedic surgery.

Whitman, Royal Am J Surg., 36: 553-57, 1937. Evolution of American orthopedic surgery.

Whitman, Royal J Bone & Joint Surg., 28: 274-77, 1946. Review of inception and development.

Whitman, Royal Proc: Royal Soc. Med., 36: 327-9, 1943. Emancipation of orthopedic surgery.

INDEX

Abbott, Leroy C.	56, 66
Albee, Fred H.	43, 56
Albert, Eduard	56
Allis, Oscar H.	56
Andry, Nicholas	14, 56
Annandale, Thomas	56
Antyllus	8
Aufranc, Otto	56
Aurelianus	8
Axhausen, Georg	23, 57
Baer, William	44
Baeyer, Hans von	57
Barlow, Thomas	57
Barton, John Rhea	29, 57
Belchier, John	57
Bell, Charles	57
Bauer, Louis	30, 57
Bick, Eugene M.	15, 57
Biesalski, Konrad	23, 45, 57
Bigelow, Henry J.	42, 58
Bircher, Eugen	58
Bleck, Eugen E.	58
Blount, Walter	58
Böhler, Thomas	58
Bohlman, Harold H.	51, 59
Borelli, Giovanni	13, 59
Brackett, E. G.	45, 59
Bradford, E. H.	59
Bristow, Rowley	59
Brodie, Benjamin	24, 59
Brown, Buckminster	37, 59
Brown, J. B.	37, 59

Buck, Gordon	59
Bunnell, Sterling	45, 59
Calot, François	60
Campbell, Willis	46, 60
Camper, Peter	14, 60
Charcot, Jean M.	60
Charnley, John	49, 60
Cheselden, William	60
Chopart, Francis	60
Chuliac, Guy de	11, 60
Codivilla, Allesandrio	61
Codman, Ernest A.	44, 61
Colles, Abraham	61
Cooper, Astley	61
Coventry, Mark	50, 61
Cunningham, J. K.	61
Davis, Gwilyn	61
Davis, H. G.	30, 31, 32, 61
daVinci, Leonardo	12
Delpech, J. M.	62
Detmold, William	30, 62
Dillehunt, R. B.	40, 62
Duchenne, G. B. A.	62
Duhamel, Henri-Louis	14, 62
Dunn, Naughton	62
Dupuytren, Guillame	62
Eikenbary, C. F.	40, 62
Elmslie, R. C.	62
Esmarch, Johann F. A. von	63
Fabrig, William	63
Fairbank, H. A. T.	22, 63
Flatt, Adrian	63
Franklin, Benjamin	28, 63
Freiberg, Albert H.	46, 63
Galen	8, 9, 10, 13

Gallie, William	63
Gibney, Virgil	32, 35, 63
Girdlestone, G.	63
Gillette, Arthur	39, 64
Glisson, Francis	64
Goldthwait, Joel	44, 64
Goodsir, John	14, 64
Guerin, J. R.	64
Hall, Marshall	64
Haller, Albrecht von	14, 64
Harrington, Paul	64
Havers, Clopton	13, 64
Henry, Arnold K.	65
Hey, William	65
Hey-Groves, Ernest W.	65
Hibbs, Russell	35, 44, 65
Hilton, John	16, 41, 65
Hippocrates	7-10
Hoffa, Albert	65
Hoffman, Phillip	65
Hoke, Michael	44, 65
Hunt, Dame Agnes	20, 65
Hunter, John	12-13, 15, 28, 41, 65-66
Hunter, William	13, 66
Ilizarov, Gavriil A.	51, 66
Insall, John	50, 66
Jansen, Mürk	66
Jones, Robert	18-21, 66
Jones, S. Fosdick	66
Judson, A. B.	33, 66
Kanavel, Allen B.	67
Keith, Arthur,	31, 67
Key, J. Albert	53, 67
Kermisson, Edouard	67
Kirkaldy-Willis	51, 52, 67

Kleinberg, Samuel	67
Knight, James	30, 32, 67
Koch, Robert	18, 67
Kocher, Emil T.	67
Küntscher, Gerhard	49, 67-68
Lambotte, Albin	68
Lane, Arbuthnot	21-22, 68
Lang, Fritz	68
Langenbeck, Bernard R. K. von	68
Leeuwenhoek, Anton van	13
Lucas-Championniere, Just	68
Leriche, Rene	68
Leveuf, Jacques	68
Lexer, Erich	24
Lister, Joseph	18, 68-69
Little, E. Muirhead	69
Little, William J.	24, 69
Long, Crawford	18
Lorenz, Adolf	23, 42, 69
Lovett, Robert	37
Macewen, William	24, 41, 69
Malgaigne, Joseph F.	69
Malphigi, Marcello	13
Mathijsen, Antonius	69
Mayer, Leo	23, 44, 45, 69
McMurray, Thomas P.	16, 69-70
Minnius, Isacius	70
Moore, Austin T.	70
Moore, James E.	39, 70
Morgan, John	37
Morris, Sir William	70
Morton, Thomas, G.	42, 70
Mott, Valentine	28, 70
Müller, M. E.	53
Murphy, John B.	70

Nelaton, Aguste	70-71
Nesbitt, Robert	71
Nichols, Edward	71
Nicola, Toufick	71
Nicoladoni, Karl	71
Ober, Frank	45, 71
Ollier, Louis X.	24, 71
Orr, H. Winnett	17, 42, 71
Osgood, Robert	71
Packard, George B.	39, 71
Paget, James	24, 72
Paracelsus	172
Paré, Ambrose	11-13, 26, 72
Park, Roswell	72
Parker, Rushton	16, 72
Pasteur, Louis	18, 72
Paul of Aegina	10
Payr, Erwin	72
Phelps, Abel	48, 73
Phelps, Winthrop M.	33, 72
Phemister, D. B.	24, 45, 73
Physick, Phillip Syng	28, 73
Platt, Sir Harry	73
Pott, Percival	14, 37, 73
Putti, Vittorio	24, 73
Recklinghausen, F. D. von	73
Redfern, Peter	73
Ridlon, John	18, 34-36, 40, 73-74
Rizzoli, Francesco	24, 74
Roentgen, Wilhelm	18, 74
Roger (King)	74
Rusk, Howard	74
Ryerson, E. W.	46, 74
Salter, Robert B.	74
Sayre, Louis	30-32, 74

Sayre, Reginald	31, 74
Schede, Max	74-75
Scudder, Charles L.	75
Sever, James	75
Shaffer, Newton	33-34, 75
Shanz, Alfred	75
Sherman, Harry	39, 75
Smith-Peterson, Marius M.	44, 75
Sprengel, Otto, G. K.	75
Starr, Clarence	76
Steele, A. J.	39, 76
Steindler, Arthur	39, 76
Steinmann, N. Fritz	76
Stoffel, Adolf	76
Stromeyer, George F. L.	24, 30, 76
Swanson, Alfred	50, 76
Sweet, John	37, 38
Syme, James	24, 76
Taylor, C. F.	30, 31, 76
Thomas, Hugh O.	16-19, 30, 34, 35, 77
Tubby, A. H.	22, 77
Velpeau, Alfred A. L. M.	77
Venel, Jean	14, 77
Vesalius, Andreas	12, 77
Volkmann, Richard von	77
Vulpius, Oscar	77
Watanabe, M.	49, 77-78
Watkins, James T.	39, 78
Watson-Jones, Sir Reginald	78
Whitman, Royal	40, 78
Willard, DeForest	78
Wilson, Harry	79
Wiltse, Leon	51, 52, 79

Would you like to see your manuscript become a book?

If you are interested in becoming a PublishAmerica author, please submit your manuscript for possible publication to us at:

acquisitions@publishamerica.com

You may also mail in your manuscript to:

**PublishAmerica
PO Box 151
Frederick, MD 21705**

www.publishamerica.com

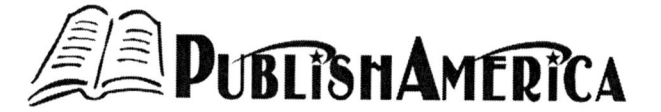

PUBLISHAMERICA